EXOCRINE PANCREATIC INSUFFICIENCY(EPI) DIET MEAL PLAN

1500+ Days recipes Reduce Inflammation and Pain Without Losing the Joy of a Tasty Meal

Aaron Sailer

Copyright © 2024

All Rights Are Reserved

The content in this book may not be reproduced, duplicated, or transferred without the express written permission of the author or publisher. Under no circumstances will the publisher or author be held liable or legally responsible for any losses, expenditures, or damages incurred directly or indirectly as a consequence of the information included in this book.

Legal Remarks

Copyright protection applies to this publication. It is only intended for personal use. No piece of this work may be modified, distributed, sold, quoted, or paraphrased without the author's or publisher's consent.

Disclaimer Statement

Please keep in mind that the contents of this booklet are meant for educational and recreational purposes. Every effort has been made to offer accurate, up-to-date, reliable, and thorough information. There are, however, no stated or implied assurances of any kind. Readers understand that the author is providing competent counsel. The content in this book originates from several sources. Please seek the opinion of a competent professional before using any of the tactics outlined in this book. By reading this book, the reader agrees that the author will not be held accountable for any direct or indirect damages resulting from the use of the information contained therein, including, but not limited to, errors, omissions, or inaccuracies.

Table of Contents

INTRODUCTION

Welcome to the delicious world of managing Exocrine Pancreatic Insufficiency (EPI) through the power of food. If you're here, chances are you or someone you care about is grappling with the complexities of EPI. Let's dive right in and demystify this condition together.

EPI, simply put, is like having a key without being able to unlock the door. Your pancreas, that hard-working organ tucked away in your abdomen, is supposed to produce digestive enzymes essential for breaking down food. But in folks with EPI, that process goes haywire. The pancreas slacks off, leaving you with a digestive system on strike and a stomach that feels like it's staging a rebellion after every meal. Sound familiar? You're not alone.

Importance of Diet in Managing EPI

Now, let's talk about the unsung hero in this tale of tummy troubles: diet. Picture your meals as the architects of your digestive destiny. What you eat can either soothe your stomach or send it into a frenzy. And when you're dealing with EPI, this becomes even more crucial.

Your body needs certain nutrients to function optimally, but with EPI in the mix, it's like playing a game of nutritional Tetris. Suddenly, you're not just thinking about what tastes good, but what your body can actually process without staging a protest. It's a delicate balancing act, but fear not – we're here to help you crack the code.

Purpose of This Book

So, why did we embark on this culinary adventure together? Well, imagine sitting at the dinner table, feeling like every bite could set off a digestive landmine. It's frustrating, disheartening, and downright exhausting. We get it.

That's where this book comes in. Consider it your trusty roadmap through the gastronomic labyrinth of EPI. Our goal? To empower you with the knowledge, tools, and mouth-watering recipes needed to take control of your digestive health and rediscover the joy of eating – sans the post-meal regret.

Throughout these pages, you'll find a treasure trove of culinary wisdom, from deciphering the intricacies of EPI to crafting personalized meal plans that nourish both body and soul. But more than just a collection of recipes, this book is a beacon of hope for anyone who's ever felt defeated by their digestive system.

CHAPTER ONE

BASICS OF EXOCRINE PANCREATIC INSUFFICIENCY

Exocrine Pancreatic Insufficiency (EPI) might sound like a mouthful, but it's essentially a digestive disorder that stems from the pancreas not producing enough digestive enzymes. Think of your pancreas as a culinary wizard – it's supposed to whip up a concoction of enzymes that help break down fats, proteins, and carbohydrates from the food you eat. But when EPI comes into play, that magical potion falls short, leaving your digestive system in disarray.

Causes and Risk Factors

Now, let's dig into the nitty-gritty of what causes this digestive hiccup. EPI can be triggered by a variety of factors, ranging from medical conditions to lifestyle choices. One of the primary culprits is chronic pancreatitis, a condition characterized by inflammation of the pancreas. Over time, this inflammation can damage the pancreatic cells responsible for producing enzymes, leading to EPI.

But chronic pancreatitis isn't the only villain in this tale. Other potential causes include cystic fibrosis, a genetic disorder that affects the pancreas and other organs, as well as pancreatic cancer, which can impede the production of digestive enzymes. Additionally, surgical procedures involving the pancreas or gastrointestinal tract can also increase the risk of developing EPI.

As for risk factors, certain demographics are more susceptible to EPI than others. Age plays a significant role, with EPI being more common in older adults due to age-related changes in pancreatic function. Individuals with a history of alcohol abuse are also at higher risk, as excessive alcohol consumption can damage the pancreas and impair enzyme production. Furthermore, smokers face an increased risk of developing EPI, as smoking has been linked to pancreas-related disorders.

Symptoms and Diagnosis

So, how do you know if EPI is knocking on your digestive door? The symptoms can vary from person to person, but there are a few tell-tale signs to watch out for. Digestive distress is a common theme, with symptoms like abdominal pain, bloating, gas, and diarrhoea making regular appearances. Unintended weight loss and malnutrition can also occur, as your body struggles to absorb nutrients properly without an adequate supply of digestive enzymes.

Diagnosing EPI can be a bit of a detective game, but your healthcare provider has a few tricks up their sleeve. Blood tests are often the first line of defence, measuring levels of certain enzymes like lipase and amylase to assess pancreatic function. Stool tests may also be conducted to check for undigested fat, a hallmark sign of EPI.

But perhaps the pièce de resistance of EPI diagnosis is the pancreatic function test, where you'll be asked to consume a meal containing a specific amount of fat, protein, and carbohydrates. Afterward, your healthcare provider will collect samples of your stool over the next few days to measure fat content and determine how effectively your body is digesting food.

In some cases, imaging tests like CT scans or MRIs may be used to evaluate the structure and function of the pancreas. And for those with underlying conditions like cystic fibrosis, genetic testing may be recommended to identify potential genetic mutations associated with EPI.

CHAPTER TWO
NUTRITIONAL REQUIREMENTS FOR EPI PATIENTS

In the intricate dance of digestion, enzymes are the unsung heroes, orchestrating the breakdown of nutrients from the foods we consume into forms our bodies can absorb and utilize. These specialized proteins act as catalysts, speeding up chemical reactions without being consumed themselves. When it comes to Exocrine Pancreatic Insufficiency (EPI), understanding the role of digestive enzymes is key to unravelling the mysteries of this digestive disorder.

Digestive enzymes are primarily produced by three organs: the pancreas, the small intestine, and the stomach. Each enzyme plays a specific role in breaking down different types of nutrients. For example, amylase helps digest carbohydrates, lipase tackles fats, and protease takes on proteins. Together, these enzymes form a formidable team, working in harmony to ensure that the nutrients from our food are properly digested and absorbed.

Now, let's zoom in on the pancreas – the powerhouse behind enzyme production. In individuals with EPI, the pancreas fails to produce an adequate number of digestive enzymes, leading to impaired digestion and nutrient malabsorption. Without enough enzymes to break down fats, proteins, and carbohydrates, undigested food particles can wreak havoc on the digestive system, causing symptoms like abdominal pain, bloating, and diarrhoea.

Key Nutrients for EPI Patients

Nutrition is the cornerstone of health – a mantra that rings especially true for individuals with Exocrine Pancreatic Insufficiency (EPI). In the delicate dance of digestive dysfunction, ensuring adequate intake of key nutrients is essential for managing symptoms, supporting overall well-being, and promoting optimal health outcomes.

So, what are these magical nutrients, and why are they so important for EPI patients? Let's break it down.

First on the list is protein – the building block of life. Protein plays a crucial role in tissue repair, immune function, and muscle maintenance. For individuals with EPI, ensuring an adequate intake of protein is essential for supporting the body's repair processes and preventing muscle wasting. Lean sources of protein, such as poultry, fish, tofu, and legumes, are generally well-tolerated and can provide a steady supply of essential amino acids without overtaxing the digestive system.

Next up, we have fats – the misunderstood macronutrient. Despite its reputation as a dietary villain, fats are actually essential for optimal health, providing energy, supporting hormone production, and aiding in the absorption of fat-soluble vitamins. However, for individuals with EPI, navigating the world of fats can be a bit trickier. Due to impaired fat digestion, high-fat foods can exacerbate symptoms like abdominal pain and diarrhoea. Opting for healthy fats from sources like avocados, nuts, seeds, and olive oil can provide the benefits of fat without the digestive distress.

And let's not forget about carbohydrates – the body's primary source of fuel. While carbohydrates often get a bad rap, they play a vital role in providing energy for daily activities and supporting brain function. For individuals with EPI, focusing on low-FODMAP carbohydrates – which are less likely to cause digestive discomfort – can help to minimize symptoms like bloating and gas. Examples of low-FODMAP carbohydrates include rice, quinoa, oats, and certain fruits and vegetables.

Recommended Daily Allowances

Navigating the world of nutritional requirements can feel like deciphering a complex code – especially for individuals with Exocrine Pancreatic Insufficiency (EPI). With digestive challenges in the mix, determining the recommended daily allowances (RDAs) for key nutrients becomes even more critical for supporting optimal health and well-being.

So, let's break it down and explore the recommended daily allowances for key nutrients, tailored specifically for individuals with EPI.

First and foremost, protein takes centre stage. As the building blocks of life, protein plays a crucial role in supporting muscle maintenance, tissue repair, and immune function. For individuals with EPI, aiming for a protein intake of 1.2 to 1.5 grams per kilogram of body weight per day is generally recommended to support optimal health and prevent muscle wasting. This translates to approximately 75 to 94 grams of protein per day for a person weighing 150 pounds.

Next up, let's talk about fats. While it's essential to be mindful of fat intake, particularly for individuals with impaired fat digestion, including healthy fats in the diet is still crucial for supporting overall health. The Institute of Medicine recommends that adults consume 20% to 35% of their daily calories from fat, with an emphasis on unsaturated fats from sources such as nuts, seeds, avocados, and olive oil. For individuals with EPI, focusing on healthy fats and incorporating enzyme supplements as needed can help to support fat digestion and absorption.

When it comes to carbohydrates, the focus shifts to quality over quantity. While there's no specific RDA for carbohydrates, aiming for a balanced diet rich in whole grains, fruits, vegetables, and legumes can provide a steady source of energy and essential nutrients. For individuals with EPI, opting for low-FODMAP carbohydrates and smaller, more frequent meals throughout the day can help to minimize digestive symptoms and support optimal digestion.

CHAPTER THREE

PRINCIPLES OF EPI DIET

In the world of nutrition, macronutrients reign supreme – these are the building blocks of our diet, providing the energy and essential nutrients our bodies need to thrive. But when it comes to managing Exocrine Pancreatic Insufficiency (EPI), striking the right balance of macronutrients becomes not just a matter of preference, but a vital component of digestive health and overall well-being.

Let's start with protein – the muscle builder and tissue repairer. Protein plays a crucial role in supporting muscle maintenance, immune function, and overall health. For individuals with EPI, ensuring an adequate intake of protein is essential for preventing muscle wasting and supporting the body's repair processes. Lean sources of protein, such as poultry, fish, tofu, and legumes, are generally well-tolerated and can provide a steady supply of essential amino acids without overtaxing the digestive system.

Next up, we have fats – the misunderstood macronutrient. Despite its reputation as a dietary villain, fats are actually essential for optimal health, providing energy, supporting hormone production, and aiding in the absorption of fat-soluble vitamins. However, for individuals with EPI, navigating the world of fats can be a bit trickier. Due to impaired fat digestion, high-fat foods can exacerbate symptoms like abdominal pain and diarrhoea. Opting for healthy fats from sources like avocados, nuts, seeds, and olive oil can provide the benefits of fat without the digestive distress.

And let's not forget about carbohydrates – the body's primary source of fuel. While carbohydrates often get a bad rap, they play a vital role in providing energy for daily activities and supporting brain function. For individuals with EPI, focusing on low-FODMAP carbohydrates – which are less likely to cause digestive discomfort – can help to minimize symptoms like bloating and gas. Examples of low-FODMAP carbohydrates include rice, quinoa, oats, and certain fruits and vegetables.

Importance of Meal Timing

Timing is everything – especially when it comes to managing Exocrine Pancreatic Insufficiency (EPI). By strategically planning meals and snacks throughout the day, individuals with EPI can optimize digestive function, minimize symptoms, and support overall health and well-being.

So, what exactly is meal timing, and why is it so important for individuals with EPI? Meal timing refers to the frequency and spacing of meals and snacks throughout the day. By eating regular, balanced meals and avoiding prolonged periods of fasting, individuals with EPI can help to regulate digestive function and prevent symptoms like bloating, gas, and abdominal discomfort.

One of the key principles of meal timing for individuals with EPI is to avoid overwhelming the digestive system with large meals or heavy snacks. Instead, opting for smaller, more frequent meals and snacks throughout the day can help to ease the burden on the pancreas and promote more efficient digestion. This approach can also help to prevent fluctuations in blood sugar levels and maintain energy levels throughout the day.

In addition to meal size and frequency, the timing of meals and snacks can also impact digestive function and symptom management. For example, eating a balanced meal or snack containing a combination of protein, healthy fats, and carbohydrates within 30 minutes to an hour of waking up can help to kick-start metabolism and provide sustained energy throughout the morning. Similarly, consuming a balanced meal or snack before bedtime can help to prevent night-time hunger and stabilize blood sugar levels.

Furthermore, paying attention to meal composition – including the types of foods consumed – can also play a role in managing symptoms of EPI. Avoiding trigger foods that exacerbate digestive symptoms, such as high-fat or high-fiber foods, can help to prevent discomfort and promote optimal digestion. Instead, opting for easily digestible foods that are rich in protein, healthy fats, and low-FODMAP carbohydrates can help to support digestive health and minimize symptoms.

Avoiding Trigger Foods

When it comes to managing Exocrine Pancreatic Insufficiency (EPI), knowledge is power – especially when it comes to identifying and avoiding trigger foods that can exacerbate symptoms and disrupt digestive function. By understanding which foods to steer clear of, individuals with EPI can take proactive steps to minimize discomfort, support optimal digestion, and promote overall well-being.

So, what exactly are trigger foods, and why are they problematic for individuals with EPI? Trigger foods are those that are known to exacerbate digestive symptoms such as bloating, gas, abdominal pain, and diarrhoea. These foods may be difficult for the digestive system to break down and can cause irritation or inflammation in the gastrointestinal tract, leading to discomfort and digestive distress.

One of the most common trigger foods for individuals with EPI is high-fat foods. Fatty foods require a significant amount of digestive enzymes to break down, and for individuals with EPI, impaired fat digestion can lead to symptoms like bloating, gas, and diarrhoea. Foods high in saturated fats, such as fried foods, fatty cuts of meat, and full-fat dairy products, should be avoided or limited to prevent digestive discomfort.

FOODS TO INCLUDE IN YOUR EPI DIET

Lean Proteins

Food Name	Portion Size	Calories	Protein (g)	Fat (g)	Carbohydrates (g)	Fiber (g)
Bison (lean cuts)	3 oz	143	22	6	0	0
Buffalo (bison) Sausage	1 link	75	14	2	0	0
Chicken or Turkey Sausage (lean)	1 link	100	12	6	1	0
Chickpeas (cooked)	1/2 cup	135	7	2	22	6
Cottage Cheese (low-fat)	1/2 cup	80	14	1	3	0
Duck Breast (skinless)	3 oz	173	30	5	0	0
Edamame (cooked)	1/2 cup	95	8	4	8	4
Eggs (boiled)	2 large	140	12	9	1	0
Elk Meat	3 oz	134	23	3	0	0
Greek Yogurt (non-fat)	6 oz	100	17	0	6	0

Kangaroo Meat	3 oz	99	22	1	0	0
Lean Beef (sirloin, tenderloin)	3 oz	155	23	6	0	0
Lean Ground Turkey	3 oz	135	21	6	0	0
Lentils (cooked)	1/2 cup	115	9	0	20	8
Ostrich Meat	3 oz	130	26	3	0	0
Pheasant	3 oz	139	28	3	0	0
Pork Tenderloin	3 oz	122	22	3	0	0
Poultry (chicken, turkey) Sausage	1 link	140	18	7	0	0
Quinoa (cooked)	1/2 cup	111	4	2	20	2
Rabbit Meat	3 oz	147	28	3	0	0
Salmon (wild-caught)	3 oz	155	22	7	0	0
Shrimp (cooked)	3 oz	90	20	1	0	0
Skinless Chicken Breast	3 oz	120	26	1	0	0
Tempeh	3 oz	160	15	9	9	0
Tofu (firm)	3 oz	70	8	4	2	1

Tuna (canned in water)	3 oz	100	22	1	0	0
Turkey Breast (cooked)	3 oz	135	26	3	0	0
Venison (deer)	3 oz	134	23	3	0	0
Venison (deer) Sausage	1 link	112	14	6	1	0
White Fish (cod, haddock, tilapia)	3 oz	90	20	1	0	0

Healthy Fats

Food Name	Portion Size	Calories	Total Fat (g)	Saturated Fat (g)	Monounsaturated Fat (g)	Polyunsaturated Fat (g)
Almonds	1/4 cup	206	18	1	11	5
Anchovies	1 oz	62	2.6	0.5	1	0.4
Avocado	1/4 medium	80	7	1	5	1
Brazil Nuts	1/4 cup	218	22	5	11	5
Cashews	1/4 cup	155	12	2	6	2
Chia Seeds	2 tablespoons	138	9	1	5	3

Coconut Flakes (unsweetened)	1/4 cup	70	7	6	1	0
Coconut Milk (canned, unsweetened)	1/4 cup	60	6	6	0	0
Coconut Oil	1 tablespoon	117	14	12	1	0
Dark Chocolate	1 oz	162	9	5	3	0
Dark Chocolate (70% cocoa or higher)	1 oz	170	12	7	4	0
Extra Firm Tofu	1/2 cup	94	5.7	1.1	2.3	2.1
Flaxseeds	2 tablespoons	75	6	1	1	5
Halibut	3 oz	140	6	1.5	2.8	1.3
Hemp Seeds	2 tablespoons	166	14	1	1	11
Herring	3 oz	100	4.8	1.2	2	1.2
Macadamia Nuts	1/4 cup	241	25	4	16	1
Mackerel	3 oz	100	6	1.8	2.2	1.3
Mussels	3 oz	70	1	0.2	0.4	0.3

Olive Oil	1 tablespoon	119	14	2	10	2	
Peanut Butter (natural)	2 tablespoons	188	16	3	8	4	
Pecans	1/4 cup	193	20	2	12	6	
Pistachios	1/4 cup	172	14	2	7	4	
Pumpkin Seeds	1/4 cup	180	15	3	4	7	
Salmon	3 oz	121	4.9	1.1	1.9	1.1	
Sardines	2 oz	100	5.1	1.4	1.3	1.8	
Sunflower Seeds	1/4 cup	204	18	1	3	11	
Tahini (sesame seed paste)	2 tablespoons	178	16	2	6	6	
Trout	3 oz	100	6	1.5	2.4	1.3	
Walnuts	1/4 cup	196	19	2	2	13	

Low-FODMAP Carbohydrates

Food Name	Portion Size	Calories	Total Carbohydrates (g)	Dietary Fiber (g)	Sugars (g)	Protein (g)	Fat (g)
Acorn Squash (cooked)	1/2 cup	32	8	2.1	1.5	0.7	0
Beetroot (cooked)	1/2 cup	37	8	1.5	6	1	0

Bell Peppers (cooked)	1/2 cup	12	3	1.1	1.6	0.5	0
Bok Choy (cooked)	1/2 cup	10	2	0.7	0.3	1	0
Buckwheat (cooked)	1/2 cup	78	17	1.5	0	3	0.6
Butternut Squash (cooked)	1/2 cup	40	10	1.5	1.5	0.9	0
Carrots (cooked)	1/2 cup	27	6	1.7	3	0.6	0
Corn (cooked)	1/2 cup	77	17	2	2	2.5	0.9
Cucumber	1/2 cup	8	2	0.3	1.5	0.3	0
Eggplant (cooked)	1/2 cup	13	3	1.7	1.8	0.5	0
Green Beans (cooked)	1/2 cup	22	5	1.9	1.9	1.3	0.1
Green Peas (cooked)	1/2 cup	62	11	3.8	4	4.1	0.4
Kale (cooked)	1/2 cup	18	4	1.4	0.6	1.3	0.3
Millet (cooked)	1/2 cup	104	22	1.7	0	3.3	0.9
Oats (rolled, cooked)	1/2 cup	83	15	1.4	0	3.2	1.4
Parsnips (cooked)	1/2 cup	55	13	3.4	3.6	0.6	0

Polenta (cooked)	1/2 cup	74	15	1.3	0	1.4	0.2
Potatoes (boiled)	1/2 cup	68	16	1.3	0	1.5	0
Pumpkin (cooked)	1/2 cup	24	6	0.5	2.5	0.6	0
Quinoa (cooked)	1/2 cup	111	20	2	0	4	1.8
Radishes	1/2 cup	9	2	1.1	1	0.4	0
Rice (white, cooked)	1/2 cup	121	26	0.4	0	2.5	0.3
Spinach (cooked)	1/2 cup	21	3	2.2	0.4	2.5	0
Sweet Potatoes (baked)	1/2 cup	90	21	3	0	2	0
Tomatoes (cooked)	1/2 cup	16	4	1.2	2.2	0.8	0
Turnips (cooked)	1/2 cup	18	4	1.3	1.8	0.5	0
Zucchini (cooked)	1/2 cup	10	2	0.6	1	0.6	0

Fiber-Rich Foods

Food Name	Portion Size	Calories	Total Carbohydrates (g)	Dietary Fiber (g)	Sugars (g)	Protein (g)
Almonds	1/4 cup	206	7	4.5	1.2	7.6

Artichokes (cooked)	1/2 cup	42	10	4.8	1.3	3.3
Black Beans (cooked)	1/2 cup	114	20	7.5	0.4	7.5
Blackberries	1/2 cup	31	7	3.5	3.5	0.6
Blueberries	1/2 cup	42	10	1.8	7	0.5
Brazil Nuts	1/4 cup	218	3	2.1	0.6	4.4
Broccoli (cooked)	1/2 cup	27	5	2.4	1.3	2.3
Brussels Sprouts	1/2 cup	28	6	2	1.3	1.8
Cashews	1/4 cup	155	9	0.9	1.7	5.1
Chia Seeds	2 tablespoons	138	12	10.6	0	4.7
Chickpeas (cooked)	1/2 cup	135	22	6.2	4.2	7.3
Collard Greens (cooked)	1/2 cup	31	5	2.7	0.5	2.3
Flaxseeds	2 tablespoons	75	4	3.8	0.3	2.6
Green Peas (cooked)	1/2 cup	62	11	3.8	4	4.1
Kale (cooked)	1/2 cup	18	4	1.4	0.6	1.3
Kidney Beans (cooked)	1/2 cup	112	20	5.7	0.3	7.7

Kiwi	1 medium	42	10	2.1	6	0.8
Lentils (cooked)	1/2 cup	115	20	7.8	0.8	9
Lima Beans (cooked)	1/2 cup	104	20	6.6	0.6	6
Oats (rolled, cooked)	1/2 cup	83	15	1.4	0	3.2
Oranges	1 medium	62	15	3	12	1.2
Pecans	1/4 cup	193	4	2.7	1.2	2.6
Pistachios	1/4 cup	172	8	2.8	2.2	6.1
Pumpkin Seeds	1/4 cup	180	4	3	0.4	9
Raspberries	1/2 cup	32	7	3.5	3.5	0.6
Spinach (cooked)	1/2 cup	21	3	2.2	0.4	2.5
Strawberries	1/2 cup	23	5	1.6	2.5	0.5
Sunflower Seeds	1/4 cup	204	7	3.9	0.7	7.3
Swiss Chard (cooked)	1/2 cup	18	3	1.7	0.4	1.5
Walnuts	1/4 cup	196	4	1.9	0.7	4.8

CHAPTER FIVE

FOODS TO AVOID

High-Fat Foods

When discussing dietary fats, it's crucial to understand that not all fats are created equal. While some fats are beneficial for health, others can have detrimental effects, especially for individuals managing Exocrine Pancreatic Insufficiency (EPI). High-fat foods are often categorized into saturated fats, trans fats, and unsaturated fats, each with its own implications for health.

- **Saturated Fats:** Saturated fats are primarily found in animal products such as meat, dairy, and eggs, as well as in certain plant-based oils like coconut and palm oil. These fats have long been associated with an increased risk of cardiovascular diseases and obesity when consumed in excess. For individuals with EPI, excessive intake of saturated fats can exacerbate symptoms due to their slow digestion and potential to increase pancreatic enzyme secretion.

- **Trans Fats:** Trans fats are primarily artificial fats created through the process of hydrogenation, often found in processed foods like margarine, fried foods, and baked goods. These fats are notorious for their adverse effects on heart health, including raising LDL (bad) cholesterol levels and increasing the risk of cardiovascular diseases. For individuals with EPI, trans fats should be strictly limited, as they can contribute to digestive discomfort and malabsorption.

- **Unsaturated Fats:** Unsaturated fats, including monounsaturated and polyunsaturated fats, are considered the healthier fats and are found in foods like nuts, seeds, avocados, and fatty fish. These fats have been shown to have beneficial effects on heart health by lowering LDL cholesterol levels and reducing inflammation. For individuals with EPI, incorporating moderate amounts of unsaturated fats into the diet can provide essential nutrients and support overall health without exacerbating symptoms.

High-Fiber Foods

Fiber is an essential nutrient that plays a crucial role in digestive health, particularly for individuals managing EPI. High-fibre foods are known for their ability to promote regular bowel movements, support gut health, and prevent constipation. However, not all types of fibre are suitable for individuals with EPI, as certain high-fibre foods may exacerbate symptoms such as bloating, gas, and diarrhoea.

- **Soluble Fiber:** Soluble fibre dissolves in water and forms a gel-like substance in the digestive tract, which helps slow down digestion and regulate blood sugar levels. Foods rich in soluble fibre include oats, legumes, nuts, seeds, and certain fruits and vegetables like apples, oranges, and carrots. For individuals with EPI, soluble fibre can be beneficial as it adds bulk to the stool and promotes regular bowel movements without causing excessive gas or bloating.

- **Insoluble Fiber:** Insoluble fibre, on the other hand, does not dissolve in water and passes through the digestive tract relatively intact, adding bulk to the stool and promoting regular bowel movements. Foods rich in insoluble fibre include whole grains, wheat bran, nuts, seeds, and certain fruits and vegetables like broccoli, cauliflower, and leafy greens. While insoluble fibre is important for overall digestive health, individuals with EPI may need to be cautious when consuming large amounts of insoluble fibre, as it can exacerbate symptoms of diarrhoea and malabsorption.

- **Bloating and Gas:** For individuals with EPI, certain high-fibre foods may contribute to symptoms of bloating and gas due to their fermentation in the colon. Foods high in fermentable fibres, such as onions, garlic, beans, and certain fruits like apples and pears, can increase gas production and lead to discomfort. It's essential for individuals with EPI to identify which high-fibre foods are well-tolerated and to consume them in moderation to minimize digestive symptoms.

Overall, incorporating a variety of high-fiber foods into the diet can provide numerous health benefits for individuals with EPI, including improved digestive health, regular bowel movements, and better management of symptoms. By choosing fiber-rich foods that are well-tolerated and avoiding those that exacerbate symptoms, individuals can optimize their dietary intake and support overall well-being.

Sugary Foods and Beverages

Sugary foods and beverages are ubiquitous in modern diets but can have detrimental effects on health, particularly for individuals managing EPI. Excessive consumption of sugar has been linked to a variety of health problems, including obesity, type 2 diabetes, and cardiovascular diseases. For individuals with EPI, high-sugar foods and beverages can exacerbate symptoms such as bloating, gas, and diarrhoea, making it essential to limit intake and prioritize healthier alternatives.

- **Effects on Blood Sugar:** Sugary foods and beverages are quickly digested and absorbed into the bloodstream, leading to rapid spikes in blood sugar levels followed by crashes. This can contribute to feelings of fatigue, irritability, and hunger, as well as long-term health problems like insulin resistance and type 2 diabetes. For individuals with EPI, managing blood sugar levels is crucial for maintaining energy levels and avoiding symptoms of hypoglycaemia.

- **Impact on Digestive Symptoms:** High-sugar foods and beverages can also exacerbate symptoms of EPI, including bloating, gas, and diarrhoea. Sugary foods like candies, pastries, and sweetened beverages contain large amounts of simple sugars that can ferment in the gut and contribute to gas production. Additionally, high-sugar diets have been associated with alterations in gut microbiota composition, which can further disrupt digestive function and exacerbate symptoms.

- **Hidden Sugars:** It's important to note that sugar can hide in unexpected places, including savoury foods like sauces, condiments, and processed snacks. Ingredients like high-fructose corn syrup, cane sugar, and maltose may be listed on food labels under different names, making it challenging to identify sources of hidden sugars. For individuals with EPI, reading food labels carefully and choosing low-sugar options can help minimize symptoms and support digestive health.

Instead of relying on sugary foods and beverages for energy, individuals with EPI can opt for healthier alternatives that provide sustained energy and essential nutrients. Whole foods like fruits, vegetables, whole grains, and lean proteins can help stabilize blood sugar levels and support overall well-being without exacerbating digestive symptoms. By prioritizing nutrient-dense foods and minimizing intake of sugary foods and beverages, individuals with EPI can optimize their dietary intake and improve their quality of life.

Processed Foods and Additives

Processed foods are a common staple in many modern diets but are often loaded with unhealthy additives, preservatives, and artificial ingredients that can have detrimental effects on health, particularly for individuals managing EPI. Processed foods are typically high in refined carbohydrates, unhealthy fats, and sodium, while lacking essential nutrients like vitamins, minerals, and fibre. For individuals with EPI, consuming processed foods can exacerbate symptoms such as bloating, gas, and diarrhoea, making it essential to limit intake and prioritize whole, unprocessed foods.

- **Effects on Digestive Health:** Processed foods often contain additives and preservatives like artificial colours, flavours, and sweeteners, as well as emulsifiers, stabilizers, and thickeners, which can disrupt digestive function and exacerbate symptoms of EPI. These additives can irritate the gastrointestinal tract, disrupt gut microbiota balance, and contribute to inflammation, leading to digestive discomfort and malabsorption. Additionally, processed foods are typically low in fibre and high in refined carbohydrates, which can further exacerbate symptoms of bloating, gas, and diarrhoea.

- **Hidden Sources of Additives:** Many processed foods contain hidden sources of additives and preservatives, making it challenging for individuals with EPI to identify and avoid them. Ingredients like monosodium glutamate (MSG), artificial sweeteners like aspartame and saccharin, and preservatives like sodium nitrate and sulphites may be lurking in processed foods like packaged snacks, frozen meals, and condiments. These additives can trigger digestive symptoms and worsen overall health, highlighting the importance of reading food labels carefully and choosing minimally processed options whenever possible.

- **Healthier Alternatives:** Instead of relying on processed foods, individuals with EPI can opt for whole, unprocessed foods that are naturally rich in nutrients and free from additives and preservatives. Fresh fruits and vegetables, whole grains, lean proteins, and healthy fats can provide essential nutrients and support digestive health without exacerbating symptoms. By prioritizing whole foods and minimizing intake of processed foods and additives, individuals with EPI can optimize their dietary intake and improve their quality of life.

CHAPTER SIX

SPECIAL CONSIDERATIONS AND MODIFICATIONS

Managing EPI in Children

Exocrine Pancreatic Insufficiency (EPI) can pose unique challenges for children, as their nutritional needs are different from those of adults, and they may have difficulty understanding and adhering to dietary restrictions. However, with proper management and support, children with EPI can lead healthy, fulfilling lives.

- **Diagnosis and Treatment:** Diagnosing EPI in children can be challenging due to the variability of symptoms and the difficulty in obtaining accurate diagnostic tests. However, early detection is crucial for preventing malnutrition and promoting growth and development. Treatment for EPI in children typically involves pancreatic enzyme replacement therapy (PERT), which helps compensate for the lack of digestive enzymes and improves nutrient absorption.

- **Nutritional Considerations:** Children with EPI may have increased energy and nutrient requirements to support growth and development. Therefore, it's essential to ensure that they receive adequate calories, protein, vitamins, and minerals through their diet. Encouraging nutrient-dense foods like fruits, vegetables, lean proteins, and whole grains can help meet these requirements while minimizing digestive symptoms.

- **Mealtime Strategies:** Mealtime can be challenging for children with EPI, as they may experience symptoms like abdominal pain, bloating, and diarrhoea after eating. It's essential to create a supportive mealtime environment and encourage positive eating behaviours, such as chewing food thoroughly and eating slowly. Additionally, offering smaller, more frequent meals and snacks throughout the day can help prevent hunger and stabilize blood sugar levels.

- **Support and Education:** Support from healthcare professionals, including paediatricians, dietitians, and gastroenterologists, is essential for managing EPI in children. Parents and caregivers should receive education and guidance on how to effectively manage their child's condition, including dietary recommendations, medication management, and symptom monitoring. Providing resources and support groups for families can also help alleviate stress and anxiety associated with managing a chronic illness.

EPI Diet for Seniors

As individuals age, their nutritional needs and digestive health can change, making it essential to tailor the EPI diet to meet the specific needs of seniors. Aging can affect digestive function, leading to a decline in pancreatic enzyme production and an increased risk of malnutrition and nutrient deficiencies. Therefore, it's crucial to optimize dietary intake and support digestive health in older adults with EPI.

- **Nutritional Needs:** Seniors with EPI may have different nutritional needs compared to younger adults due to age-related changes in metabolism, digestion, and nutrient absorption. Therefore, it's essential to ensure that they receive adequate calories, protein, vitamins, and minerals to support overall health and well-being. Encouraging nutrient-dense foods like lean proteins, fruits, vegetables, and whole grains can help meet these requirements while minimizing digestive symptoms.

- **Mealtime Challenges:** Seniors with EPI may experience mealtime challenges such as poor appetite, difficulty chewing or swallowing, and gastrointestinal symptoms like bloating, gas, and diarrhoea. It's essential to address these issues and provide support and accommodations to make mealtime more enjoyable and manageable. This may include offering smaller, more frequent meals, adapting textures and consistencies to facilitate swallowing, and providing assistance with meal preparation and feeding as needed.

- **Medication Management:** Seniors with EPI may be taking multiple medications for various health conditions, which can interact with pancreatic enzyme replacement therapy (PERT) and affect nutrient absorption. It's essential to monitor medication use carefully and adjust PERT dosages accordingly to ensure optimal digestion and nutrient absorption. Healthcare professionals should review medication regimens regularly and make adjustments as needed to minimize gastrointestinal symptoms and optimize nutritional status.

- **Hydration and Fluid Intake:** Seniors are at increased risk of dehydration due to age-related changes in thirst perception, kidney function, and fluid balance. Therefore, it's essential to encourage adequate hydration and fluid intake to prevent constipation, urinary tract infections, and other complications. Offering fluids with meals and snacks, such as water, herbal teas, and broth-based soups, can help seniors meet their fluid needs and support overall digestive health.

Adjusting the Diet for Weight Management

Weight management is an important aspect of managing Exocrine Pancreatic Insufficiency (EPI), as excess body weight can exacerbate symptoms and increase the risk of complications such as diabetes, heart disease, and digestive problems. Therefore, adjusting the diet to achieve and maintain a healthy weight is essential for individuals with EPI.

- **Caloric Intake:** Achieving a healthy weight involves balancing caloric intake with energy expenditure to create a calorie deficit or surplus, depending on weight loss or weight gain goals. For individuals with EPI, it's important to monitor caloric intake carefully and adjust portion sizes and meal frequency as needed to achieve and maintain a healthy weight. Working with a registered dietitian can help develop personalized meal plans that meet individual calorie needs while supporting overall health and well-being.

- **Macronutrient Balance:** In addition to monitoring caloric intake, it's essential to pay attention to macronutrient balance, including carbohydrates, protein, and fat. For individuals with EPI, focusing on nutrient-dense foods like fruits, vegetables, lean proteins, and whole grains can help promote satiety, stabilize blood sugar levels, and support weight management goals. Avoiding high-fat and high-sugar foods that contribute excess calories without providing essential nutrients can also help prevent weight gain and improve overall health.

- **Physical Activity:** Physical activity plays a crucial role in weight management and overall health for individuals with EPI. Regular exercise helps burn calories, build muscle mass, and improve metabolic function, all of which contribute to maintaining a healthy weight. Encouraging activities like walking, cycling, swimming, and strength training can help individuals with EPI stay active and achieve their weight management goals.

- **Behavioural Strategies:** Achieving and maintaining a healthy weight requires adopting healthy eating and lifestyle habits that promote long-term success. This may include mindful eating practices, such as paying attention to hunger and fullness cues, practicing portion control, and avoiding emotional eating. Additionally, setting realistic goals, tracking progress, and seeking support from healthcare professionals and support groups can help individuals with EPI stay motivated and on track with their weight management efforts.

CHAPTER SEVEN

LIFESTYLE STRATEGIES FOR MANAGING EPI

Stress Management Techniques

Stress is an inevitable part of life, but when it becomes chronic or overwhelming, it can have serious implications for both physical and mental health. For individuals managing Exocrine Pancreatic Insufficiency (EPI), stress management is particularly important, as stress can exacerbate digestive symptoms and impact overall well-being. Fortunately, there are several effective techniques for managing stress and promoting a sense of calm and balance.

- **Mindfulness Meditation:** Mindfulness meditation involves paying attention to the present moment without judgment, which can help reduce stress and increase feelings of relaxation and well-being. Practicing mindfulness meditation regularly can help individuals with EPI cultivate a greater sense of awareness and acceptance of their thoughts, feelings, and bodily sensations, allowing them to respond to stressors more effectively and with greater resilience.

- **Deep Breathing Exercises:** Deep breathing exercises, such as diaphragmatic breathing or belly breathing, can help activate the body's relaxation response and reduce stress and anxiety. By taking slow, deep breaths and focusing on the sensation of air entering and leaving the body, individuals with EPI can calm their nervous system, lower their heart rate, and promote feelings of relaxation and tranquillity.

- **Progressive Muscle Relaxation:** Progressive muscle relaxation involves tensing and then relaxing different muscle groups throughout the body, which can help release tension and reduce physical symptoms of stress. By systematically tensing and releasing muscle groups from head to toe, individuals with EPI can promote relaxation and alleviate muscle tension, allowing them to feel more at ease and less stressed.

- **Cognitive-Behavioural Therapy (CBT):** Cognitive-behavioural therapy is a type of psychotherapy that focuses on identifying and challenging negative thought patterns and behaviours that contribute to stress and anxiety. By learning to reframe negative thoughts and develop more adaptive coping strategies, individuals with EPI can reduce stress and improve their ability to manage challenging situations effectively.

- **Healthy Lifestyle Habits:** In addition to specific stress management techniques, adopting healthy lifestyle habits can also help individuals with EPI better cope with stress and promote overall well-being. This includes getting regular exercise, eating a balanced diet, getting enough sleep, and engaging in activities that bring joy and fulfilment.

In conclusion, stress management is essential for individuals managing Exocrine Pancreatic Insufficiency (EPI) to promote overall well-being and minimize the impact of stress on digestive symptoms. By incorporating mindfulness meditation, deep breathing exercises, progressive muscle relaxation, cognitive-behavioural therapy, and healthy lifestyle habits into their routine, individuals with EPI can effectively manage stress and improve their quality of life.

Exercise Recommendations

Regular physical activity is essential for overall health and well-being, including for individuals managing Exocrine Pancreatic Insufficiency (EPI). Exercise not only helps maintain a healthy weight and improve cardiovascular health but can also support digestive function and reduce stress and anxiety. Here are some exercise recommendations for individuals with EPI to consider:

- **Aerobic Exercise:** Aerobic exercise, also known as cardiovascular exercise, involves activities that increase heart rate and breathing rate, such as walking, jogging, cycling, swimming, and dancing. Aerobic exercise helps improve cardiovascular health, boost metabolism, and increase energy levels, all of which can benefit individuals with EPI. Aim for at least 150 minutes of moderate-intensity aerobic exercise or 75 minutes of vigorous-intensity aerobic exercise per week, as recommended by the American Heart Association.

- **Strength Training:** Strength training, also known as resistance training, involves activities that strengthen muscles and bones, such as lifting weights, using resistance bands, or performing bodyweight exercises. Strength training helps build lean muscle mass, improve bone density, and increase metabolism, all of which can support overall health and well-being. Aim to include strength training exercises at least two days per week, targeting major muscle groups like the legs, arms, chest, back, and core.

- **Flexibility and Balance Exercises:** Flexibility and balance exercises help improve range of motion, joint mobility, and stability, reducing the risk of falls and injuries, particularly in older adults with EPI. Activities like yoga, Pilates, tai chi, and stretching can help improve flexibility, balance, and coordination, promoting overall physical function and well-being. Aim to incorporate flexibility and balance exercises into your routine at least two to three days per week, focusing on stretching major muscle groups and practicing balance poses and movements.

- **Low-Impact Activities:** For individuals with EPI who may experience digestive discomfort or joint pain during high-impact activities, low-impact exercises like swimming, cycling, walking, and elliptical training can provide an effective alternative. These activities are gentle on the joints and can be easily modified to suit individual fitness levels and preferences, making them ideal for individuals with EPI looking to stay active and maintain their health.

- **Listen to Your Body:** When engaging in exercise, it's essential to listen to your body and pay attention to how you feel. If you experience any pain, discomfort, or fatigue, it's important to stop and rest or modify your activities accordingly. Gradually increase the intensity, duration, and frequency of your workouts over time, allowing your body to adapt and progress safely.

Importance of Hydration

Proper hydration is essential for overall health and well-being, including for individuals managing Exocrine Pancreatic Insufficiency (EPI). Water plays a crucial role in digestion, nutrient absorption, temperature regulation, and waste elimination, making it essential for optimal digestive function and overall health. Here are some reasons why hydration is important for individuals with EPI:

- **Digestive Function:** Water is essential for proper digestion and nutrient absorption, as it helps break down food particles, lubricate the digestive tract, and facilitate the movement of waste through the intestines. Adequate hydration can help prevent constipation, promote regular bowel movements, and alleviate symptoms of digestive discomfort associated with EPI.

- **Pancreatic Enzyme Activation:** Proper hydration is necessary for the activation and function of pancreatic enzymes, which are essential for breaking down carbohydrates, proteins, and fats in the digestive tract. Without adequate hydration, pancreatic enzyme activity may be impaired, leading to poor digestion and nutrient malabsorption, particularly in individuals with EPI.

- **Regulation of Body Temperature:** Water plays a crucial role in regulating body temperature, especially during physical activity and in hot or humid environments. Proper hydration helps maintain electrolyte balance and prevents dehydration, heat exhaustion, and heatstroke, all of which can negatively impact digestive function and overall health, particularly in individuals with EPI.

- **Cognitive Function:** Hydration is essential for optimal cognitive function, including memory, concentration, and mood regulation. Dehydration can impair cognitive performance and lead to feelings of fatigue, irritability, and difficulty focusing, all of which can impact daily functioning and quality of life, particularly in individuals with EPI.

- **Symptom Management:** Proper hydration can help alleviate symptoms associated with EPI, such as bloating, gas, and diarrhoea, by promoting regular bowel movements, flushing out toxins and waste products, and supporting overall digestive health. Drinking plenty of water throughout the day can help keep digestive symptoms at bay and improve overall well-being.

BREAKFAST RECIPES

Scrambled Tofu Breakfast Tacos

Ingredients:

- 1 tablespoon olive oil

- 1 block (14 oz.) firm tofu, drained and crumbled

- 1 bell pepper, diced

- 1 small onion, diced

- 2 cloves garlic, minced

- 1 teaspoon ground cumin

- 1 teaspoon chili powder

- Salt and pepper to taste

- 4 whole grain or corn tortillas

- Salsa, avocado, and cilantro for serving

Prep Time: 10 mins

Cooking Time: 10 mins

Total Time: 20 mins

Servings: 4

Nutrition Facts (per serving):

- Calories: 215

- Fat: 10g

- Saturated fat: 1g

- Cholesterol: 0mg

- Sodium: 247mg

- Carbohydrate: 22g

- Fiber: 5g

- Sugar: 4g

- Protein: 11g

- Calcium: 126mg

- Iron: 2mg

Instructions:

1. Heat olive oil in a skillet over medium heat. Add diced bell pepper and onion, and sauté until softened, about 5 minutes.

2. Add minced garlic to the skillet and cook for another minute.

3. Stir in crumbled tofu, ground cumin, chili powder, salt, and pepper. Cook for 3-4 minutes, stirring occasionally, until tofu is heated through.

4. Warm tortillas in a separate skillet or in the microwave.

5. Spoon tofu mixture onto tortillas, and top with salsa, sliced avocado, and chopped cilantro.

6. Serve immediately and enjoy your delicious scrambled tofu breakfast tacos!

Banana Oatmeal Pancakes

Ingredients:

- 2 ripe bananas, mashed

- 2 eggs

- 1 cup rolled oats

- 1 teaspoon baking powder

- 1/2 teaspoon ground cinnamon

- 1/4 teaspoon salt

- 1/4 cup milk (or almond milk)

- 1 tablespoon honey (optional)

- Cooking spray or butter for greasing the skillet

Prep Time: 10 mins

Cooking Time: 10 mins

Total Time: 20 mins

Servings: 4 (3 pancakes per serving)

Nutrition Facts (per serving):

- Calories: 204

- Fat: 5g

- Saturated fat: 1g

- Cholesterol: 107mg

- Sodium: 316mg

- Carbohydrate: 34g

- Fiber: 4g

- Sugar: 10g

- Protein: 8g

- Calcium: 101mg

- Iron: 2mg

Instructions:

1. In a large mixing bowl, combine mashed bananas, eggs, rolled oats, baking powder, ground cinnamon, salt, milk, and honey (if using). Mix until well combined.

2. Heat a non-stick skillet or griddle over medium heat and lightly grease with cooking spray or butter.

3. Pour about 1/4 cup of pancake batter onto the skillet for each pancake. Cook until bubbles form on the surface, then flip and cook until golden brown on both sides.

4. Repeat with the remaining batter, greasing the skillet as needed.

5. Serve warm with your favourite toppings such as fresh fruit, yogurt, or maple syrup.

6. Enjoy these nutritious and delicious banana oatmeal pancakes for a satisfying breakfast!

Veggie and Egg Breakfast Burrito

Ingredients:

- 4 large eggs

- 1 tablespoon olive oil

- 1 bell pepper, diced

- 1 small onion, diced

- 1 cup sliced mushrooms

- 1 cup spinach leaves

- Salt and pepper to taste

- 4 whole grain or spinach tortillas

- Salsa and avocado for serving

Prep Time: 10 mins

Cooking Time: 10 mins

Total Time: 20 mins

Servings: 4

Nutrition Facts (per serving):

- Calories: 225

- Fat: 11g

- Saturated fat: 2g

- Cholesterol: 186mg

- Sodium: 245mg

- Carbohydrate: 21g

- Fiber: 4g

- Sugar: 4g

- Protein: 11g

- Calcium: 88mg

- Iron: 2mg

Instructions:

1. In a large skillet, heat olive oil over medium heat. Add diced bell pepper, onion, and mushrooms, and sauté until softened, about 5 minutes.

2. Add spinach leaves to the skillet and cook until wilted, about 2 minutes. Season with salt and pepper to taste.

3. In a separate bowl, beat eggs and pour into the skillet with the cooked vegetables. Cook, stirring occasionally, until eggs are scrambled and cooked through.

4. Warm tortillas in a separate skillet or in the microwave.

5. Divide the egg and vegetable mixture evenly among the tortillas. Top with salsa and sliced avocado.

6. Roll up the tortillas, folding in the sides, to form burritos.

7. Serve immediately and enjoy your nutritious and flavourful veggie and egg breakfast burritos!

Greek Yogurt Parfait

Ingredients:

- 1 cup Greek yogurt

- 1/2 cup granola

- 1/2 cup mixed berries (such as strawberries, blueberries, and raspberries)

- 1 tablespoon honey (optional)

- 1 tablespoon chopped nuts (such as almonds or walnuts)

Prep Time: 5 mins

Total Time: 5 mins

Servings: 1

Nutrition Facts (per serving):

- Calories: 320

- Fat: 9g

- Saturated fat: 1g

- Cholesterol: 10mg

- Sodium: 60mg

- Carbohydrate: 45g

- Fiber: 6g

- Sugar: 22g

- Protein: 17g

- Calcium: 150mg

- Iron: 2mg

Instructions:

1. In a serving glass or bowl, layer Greek yogurt, granola, and mixed berries.

2. Drizzle honey over the top for added sweetness, if desired.

3. Sprinkle chopped nuts over the parfait for added crunch and flavor.

4. Serve immediately and enjoy this delicious and nutritious Greek yogurt parfait for a quick and easy breakfast option!

Avocado Toast with Poached Egg

Ingredients:

- 2 slices whole grain bread

- 1 ripe avocado

- 2 large eggs

- Salt and pepper to taste

- Red pepper flakes (optional)

- Fresh herbs (such as parsley or cilantro) for garnish

Prep Time: 5 mins

Cooking Time: 5 mins

Total Time: 10 mins

Servings: 2

Nutrition Facts (per serving):

- Calories: 290

- Fat: 17g

- Saturated fat: 3g

- Cholesterol: 186mg

- Sodium: 250mg

- Carbohydrate: 23g

- Fiber: 8g

- Sugar: 2g

- Protein: 13g

- Calcium: 54mg

- Iron: 2mg

Instructions:

1. Toast the slices of whole grain bread until golden brown.

2. While the bread is toasting, mash the ripe avocado in a small bowl and season with salt and pepper to taste.

3. Poach the eggs: Bring a pot of water to a simmer and carefully crack the eggs into the simmering water. Cook for about 3-4 minutes until the egg whites are set but the yolks are still runny. Remove with a slotted spoon and drain on a paper towel.

4. Spread the mashed avocado evenly onto the toasted bread slices.

5. Place a poached egg on top of each avocado toast.

6. Season with additional salt, pepper, and red pepper flakes if desired.

7. Garnish with fresh herbs for added flavor and visual appeal.

8. Serve immediately and enjoy your delicious and nutritious avocado toast with poached egg for a satisfying breakfast!

Quinoa Breakfast Bowl

Ingredients:

- 1/2 cup cooked quinoa

- 1/4 cup sliced almonds

- 1/4 cup fresh berries (such as strawberries, blueberries, or raspberries)

- 1 tablespoon honey or maple syrup (optional)

- 1/2 teaspoon ground cinnamon

- 1/4 cup Greek yogurt

Prep Time: 5 mins

Cooking Time: 15 mins (for cooking quinoa)

Total Time: 20 mins

Servings: 1

Nutrition Facts (per serving):

- Calories: 300

- Fat: 10g

- Saturated fat: 1g

- Cholesterol: 2mg

- Sodium: 25mg

- Carbohydrate: 45g

- Fiber: 6g

- Sugar: 14g

- Protein: 12g

- Calcium: 100mg

- Iron: 3mg

Instructions:

1. Cook quinoa according to package instructions.

2. In a serving bowl, layer cooked quinoa, sliced almonds, and fresh berries.

3. Drizzle honey or maple syrup over the top, if desired, and sprinkle ground cinnamon.

4. Top with Greek yogurt.

5. Serve immediately and enjoy this nutritious and delicious quinoa breakfast bowl!

Spinach and Feta Omelette

Ingredients:

- 2 large eggs

- 1 tablespoon milk (or almond milk)

- Salt and pepper to taste

- 1/2 cup fresh spinach leaves

- 2 tablespoons crumbled feta cheese

- 1 teaspoon olive oil

Prep Time: 5 mins

Cooking Time: 5 mins

Total Time: 10 mins

Servings: 1

Nutrition Facts (per serving):

- Calories: 240

- Fat: 18g

- Saturated fat: 6g

- Cholesterol: 372mg

- Sodium: 520mg

- Carbohydrate: 2g

- Fiber: 0g

- Sugar: 1g

- Protein: 16g

- Calcium: 171mg

- Iron: 2mg

Instructions:

1. In a bowl, whisk together eggs, milk, salt, and pepper.

2. Heat olive oil in a non-stick skillet over medium heat. Add spinach leaves and cook until wilted.

3. Pour the egg mixture into the skillet, swirling to evenly distribute.

4. Cook until the edges begin to set, then sprinkle crumbled feta cheese over one half of the omelette.

5. Fold the other half of the omelette over the filling and cook for another minute until the cheese melts and the eggs are cooked through.

6. Slide the omelette onto a plate and serve immediately.

7. Enjoy this spinach and feta omelette for a protein-packed breakfast option!

Chia Seed Pudding

Ingredients:

- 1/4 cup chia seeds

- 1 cup unsweetened almond milk (or any milk of choice)

- 1 tablespoon honey or maple syrup (optional)

- 1/2 teaspoon vanilla extract

- Fresh fruit for topping (such as berries or sliced bananas)

- Nuts or seeds for topping (such as almonds or pumpkin seeds)

Prep Time: 5 mins

Total Time: 4 hours (for chilling)

Servings: 2

Nutrition Facts (per serving):

- Calories: 180

- Fat: 9g

- Saturated fat: 1g

- Cholesterol: 0mg

- Sodium: 85mg

- Carbohydrate: 20g

- Fiber: 10g

- Sugar: 7g

- Protein: 5g

- Calcium: 400mg

- Iron: 3mg

Instructions:

1. In a bowl, combine chia seeds, almond milk, honey or maple syrup (if using), and vanilla extract. Stir well to combine.

2. Cover the bowl and refrigerate for at least 4 hours or overnight, until the chia pudding has thickened.

3. Stir the chia pudding before serving, and divide into serving bowls.

4. Top with fresh fruit and nuts or seeds.

5. Serve chilled and enjoy this creamy and nutritious chia seed pudding for breakfast!

Sweet Potato Hash

Ingredients:

- 1 large sweet potato, peeled and diced

- 1/2 bell pepper, diced

- 1/2 onion, diced

- 2 cloves garlic, minced

- 2 tablespoons olive oil

- 1 teaspoon smoked paprika

- Salt and pepper to taste

- Fresh parsley for garnish

Prep Time: 10 mins

Cooking Time: 20 mins

Total Time: 30 mins

Servings: 2

Nutrition Facts (per serving):

- Calories: 230

- Fat: 14g

- Saturated fat: 2g

- Cholesterol: 0mg

- Sodium: 65mg

- Carbohydrate: 25g

- Fiber: 4g

- Sugar: 6g

- Protein: 2g

- Vitamin C: 40mg

- Iron: 1mg

Instructions:

1. Heat olive oil in a skillet over medium heat. Add diced sweet potato and cook until tender, about 10 minutes.

2. Add diced bell pepper, onion, and minced garlic to the skillet. Cook until vegetables are softened, about 5 minutes.

3. Season the hash with smoked paprika, salt, and pepper, stirring to combine.

4. Continue cooking for another 5 minutes, until the sweet potatoes are caramelized and the vegetables are cooked through.

5. Garnish with fresh parsley and serve hot.

6. Enjoy this flavourful and nutritious sweet potato hash for a satisfying breakfast option!

Blueberry Almond Overnight Oats

Ingredients:

- 1/2 cup rolled oats

- 1/2 cup unsweetened almond milk (or any milk of choice)

- 1/4 cup Greek yogurt

- 1 tablespoon almond butter

- 1 tablespoon honey or maple syrup

- 1/4 cup fresh blueberries

- 1 tablespoon sliced almonds

Prep Time: 5 mins

Total Time: 8 hours (for chilling overnight)

Servings: 1

Nutrition Facts (per serving):

- Calories: 330

- Fat: 12g

- Saturated fat: 1g

- Cholesterol: 2mg

- Sodium: 85mg

- Carbohydrate: 45g

- Fiber: 7g

- Sugar: 17g

- Protein: 11g

- Calcium: 300mg

- Iron: 2mg

Instructions:

1. In a jar or container, combine rolled oats, almond milk, Greek yogurt, almond butter, and honey or maple syrup. Stir well to combine.

2. Gently fold in fresh blueberries.

3. Cover the jar or container and refrigerate overnight, or for at least 8 hours.

4. In the morning, stir the overnight oats and top with sliced almonds.

5. Enjoy these delicious and convenient blueberry almond overnight oats for a quick and nutritious breakfast option!

Smoked Salmon Avocado Toast

Ingredients:

- 2 slices whole grain bread, toasted

- 1/2 ripe avocado, mashed

- 2 oz. smoked salmon

- 1 tablespoon capers

- Fresh dill for garnish

- Lemon wedges for serving

Prep Time: 5 mins

Total Time: 5 mins

Servings: 1

Nutrition Facts (per serving):

- Calories: 280

- Fat: 15g

- Saturated fat: 2g

- Cholesterol: 15mg

- Sodium: 670mg

- Carbohydrate: 23g

- Fiber: 7g

- Sugar: 1g

- Protein: 17g

- Calcium: 52mg

- Iron: 2mg

Instructions:

1. Spread mashed avocado evenly onto toasted whole grain bread slices.

2. Top with smoked salmon slices.

3. Sprinkle capers over the salmon.

4. Garnish with fresh dill.

5. Serve with lemon wedges on the side.

6. Enjoy this flavourful and nutritious smoked salmon avocado toast for breakfast!

Veggie Frittata

Ingredients:

- 6 large eggs

- 1/4 cup milk (or almond milk)

- 1/2 cup diced bell peppers

- 1/2 cup diced onions

- 1/2 cup diced tomatoes

- 1/2 cup chopped spinach

- Salt and pepper to taste

- 1 tablespoon olive oil

Prep Time: 10 mins

Cooking Time: 20 mins

Total Time: 30 mins

Servings: 4

Nutrition Facts (per serving):

- Calories: 150

- Fat: 10g

- Saturated fat: 2g

- Cholesterol: 280mg

- Sodium: 160mg

- Carbohydrate: 6g

- Fiber: 1g

- Sugar: 3g

- Protein: 10g

- Calcium: 52mg

- Iron: 1mg

Instructions:

1. Preheat oven to 350°F (175°C).

2. In a bowl, whisk together eggs, milk, salt, and pepper.

3. Heat olive oil in an oven-safe skillet over medium heat. Add diced bell peppers and onions, and sauté until softened.

4. Add diced tomatoes and chopped spinach to the skillet, and cook until spinach wilts.

5. Pour the egg mixture evenly over the vegetables in the skillet.

6. Cook for a few minutes until the edges begin to set.

7. Transfer the skillet to the preheated oven and bake for 15-20 minutes, until the frittata is set and golden brown on top.

8. Slice into wedges and serve hot.

9. Enjoy this delicious and nutrient-packed veggie frittata for a satisfying breakfast!

Apple Cinnamon Overnight Oats

Ingredients:

- 1/2 cup rolled oats

- 1/2 cup unsweetened almond milk (or any milk of choice)

- 1/4 cup Greek yogurt

- 1/2 apple, diced

- 1 tablespoon honey or maple syrup

- 1/2 teaspoon ground cinnamon

- 1 tablespoon chopped walnuts

Prep Time: 5 mins

Total Time: 8 hours (for chilling overnight)

Servings: 1

Nutrition Facts (per serving):

- Calories: 320

- Fat: 10g

- Saturated fat: 1g

- Cholesterol: 2mg

- Sodium: 85mg

- Carbohydrate: 50g

- Fiber: 7g

- Sugar: 21g

- Protein: 10g

- Calcium: 250mg

- Iron: 2mg

Instructions:

1. In a jar or container, combine rolled oats, almond milk, Greek yogurt, diced apple, honey or maple syrup, ground cinnamon, and chopped walnuts. Stir well to combine.

2. Cover the jar or container and refrigerate overnight, or for at least 8 hours.

3. In the morning, stir the overnight oats and serve chilled.

4. Enjoy this delicious and nutritious apple cinnamon overnight oats for a convenient breakfast option!

Turkey and Veggie Breakfast Wrap

Ingredients:

- 1 whole grain or spinach tortilla

- 2 slices turkey breast

- 1/4 cup diced bell peppers

- 1/4 cup diced onions

- 1/4 cup chopped spinach

- 1 tablespoon salsa

- Salt and pepper to taste

Prep Time: 5 mins

Cooking Time: 5 mins

Total Time: 10 mins

Servings: 1

Nutrition Facts (per serving):

- Calories: 180

- Fat: 5g

- Saturated fat: 1g

- Cholesterol: 25mg

- Sodium: 520mg

- Carbohydrate: 18g

- Fiber: 3g

- Sugar: 3g

- Protein: 15g

- Calcium: 40mg

- Iron: 1mg

Instructions:

1. Heat a skillet over medium heat. Place the tortilla on the skillet and warm for about 30 seconds on each side.

2. Layer turkey breast slices on the tortilla.

3. In the same skillet, add diced bell peppers and onions, and sauté until softened.

4. Add chopped spinach to the skillet and cook until wilted.

5. Season with salt and pepper to taste.

6. Spoon the cooked vegetables over the turkey slices.

7. Drizzle salsa over the top.

8. Roll up the tortilla to form a wrap.

9. Serve immediately and enjoy this protein-packed turkey and veggie breakfast wrap!

Cottage Cheese and Fruit Bowl

Ingredients:

- 1/2 cup low-fat cottage cheese

- 1/2 cup mixed fresh fruit (such as berries, sliced banana, and diced apple)

- 1 tablespoon chopped nuts (such as almonds or walnuts)

- 1 teaspoon honey or maple syrup (optional)

Prep Time: 5 mins

Total Time: 5 mins

Servings: 1

Nutrition Facts (per serving):

- Calories: 210

- Fat: 6g

- Saturated fat: 1g

- Cholesterol: 10mg

- Sodium: 400mg

- Carbohydrate: 24g

- Fiber: 4g

- Sugar: 16g

- Protein: 16g

- Calcium: 100mg

- Iron: 1mg

Instructions:

1. In a bowl, spoon low-fat cottage cheese.

2. Top with mixed fresh fruit.

3. Sprinkle chopped nuts over the fruit.

4. Drizzle honey or maple syrup over the top, if desired.

5. Serve immediately and enjoy this simple and nutritious cottage cheese and fruit bowl for a refreshing breakfast option!

LUNCH RECIPES

Grilled Lemon Herb Chicken Salad

Ingredients:

- 2 boneless, skinless chicken breasts

- 2 tablespoons olive oil

- 2 cloves garlic, minced

- Zest and juice of 1 lemon

- 1 teaspoon dried oregano

- 1 teaspoon dried thyme

- Salt and pepper to taste

- 4 cups mixed salad greens

- 1 cup cherry tomatoes, halved

- 1/2 cucumber, sliced

- 1/4 cup crumbled feta cheese

- 2 tablespoons balsamic vinaigrette

Prep Time: 10 mins

Cooking Time: 12 mins

Total Time: 22 mins

Servings: 2

Nutrition Facts (per serving):

- Calories: 320

- Fat: 16g

- Saturated fat: 4g

- Cholesterol: 90mg

- Sodium: 420mg

- Carbohydrate: 10g

- Fiber: 3g

- Sugar: 4g

- Protein: 34g

- Vitamin C: 30mg

- Calcium: 150mg

- Iron: 2mg

Instructions:

1. Preheat grill to medium-high heat.

2. In a small bowl, whisk together olive oil, minced garlic, lemon zest, lemon juice, dried oregano, dried thyme, salt, and pepper.

3. Place chicken breasts in a shallow dish and pour the marinade over them. Allow to marinate for at least 10 minutes.

4. Grill chicken breasts for about 6 minutes per side, or until cooked through and no longer pink in the centre.

5. Remove chicken from grill and let rest for a few minutes before slicing.

6. In a large bowl, toss mixed salad greens, cherry tomatoes, cucumber slices, and crumbled feta cheese.

7. Divide the salad mixture between two plates and top with sliced grilled chicken.

8. Drizzle with balsamic vinaigrette dressing.

9. Serve immediately and enjoy this refreshing and nutritious grilled lemon herb chicken salad!

Quinoa Salad with Roasted Vegetables

Ingredients:

- 1 cup quinoa, rinsed

- 2 cups water or vegetable broth

- 1 red bell pepper, diced

- 1 yellow bell pepper, diced

- 1 zucchini, diced

- 1 red onion, diced

- 2 tablespoons olive oil

- 1 teaspoon dried thyme

- 1 teaspoon dried rosemary

- Salt and pepper to taste

- 1/4 cup chopped fresh parsley

- 1/4 cup crumbled goat cheese (optional)

- Balsamic vinaigrette dressing for serving

Prep Time: 10 mins

Cooking Time: 25 mins

Total Time: 35 mins

Servings: 4

Nutrition Facts (per serving):

- Calories: 290

- Fat: 11g

- Saturated fat: 2g

- Cholesterol: 5mg

- Sodium: 80mg

- Carbohydrate: 38g

- Fiber: 6g

- Sugar: 4g

- Protein: 9g

- Vitamin C: 70mg

- Calcium: 80mg

- Iron: 3mg

Instructions:

1. Preheat oven to 400°F (200°C).

2. In a medium saucepan, combine quinoa and water or vegetable broth. Bring to a boil, then reduce heat, cover, and simmer for 15-20 minutes, or until quinoa is cooked and water is absorbed. Fluff with a fork and set aside.

3. Meanwhile, spread diced bell peppers, zucchini, and red onion on a baking sheet. Drizzle with olive oil and sprinkle with dried thyme, dried rosemary, salt, and pepper. Toss to coat evenly.

4. Roast vegetables in the preheated oven for 20-25 minutes, or until tender and lightly browned, stirring halfway through.

5. In a large bowl, combine cooked quinoa, roasted vegetables, chopped parsley, and crumbled goat cheese (if using). Toss gently to combine.

6. Serve quinoa salad with roasted vegetables at room temperature or chilled, drizzled with balsamic vinaigrette dressing.

7. Enjoy this flavourful and satisfying quinoa salad as a healthy lunch option!

Turkey and Avocado Wrap

Ingredients:

- 2 whole grain or spinach tortillas

- 4 slices turkey breast

- 1 avocado, sliced

- 1/2 cup baby spinach leaves

- 1/4 cup shredded carrots

- 2 tablespoons hummus

Prep Time: 5 mins

Total Time: 5 mins

Servings: 2

Nutrition Facts (per serving):

- Calories: 280

- Fat: 14g

- Saturated fat: 2g

- Cholesterol: 35mg

- Sodium: 560mg

- Carbohydrate: 24g

- Fiber: 7g

- Sugar: 1g

- Protein: 17g

- Vitamin C: 15mg

- Calcium: 70mg

- Iron: 2mg

Instructions:

1. Lay out tortillas on a clean work surface.

2. Spread 1 tablespoon of hummus evenly over each tortilla.

3. Layer turkey breast slices, avocado slices, baby spinach leaves, and shredded carrots evenly over each tortilla.

4. Roll up the tortillas tightly to form wraps.

5. Slice each wrap in half diagonally.

6. Serve immediately and enjoy these delicious and nutritious turkey and avocado wraps for lunch!

Lentil and Vegetable Soup

Ingredients:

- 1 tablespoon olive oil

- 1 onion, diced

- 2 carrots, diced

- 2 celery stalks, diced

- 2 cloves garlic, minced

- 1 cup dried green lentils, rinsed

- 4 cups vegetable broth

- 1 bay leaf

- 1 teaspoon dried thyme

- Salt and pepper to taste

- 2 tablespoons chopped fresh parsley

- Lemon wedges for serving

Prep Time: 10 mins

Cooking Time: 30 mins

Total Time: 40 mins

Servings: 4

Nutrition Facts (per serving):

- Calories: 230

- Fat: 4g

- Saturated fat: 0.5g

- Cholesterol: 0mg

- Sodium: 580mg

- Carbohydrate: 38g

- Fiber: 15g

- Sugar: 6g

- Protein: 12g

- Vitamin C: 10mg

- Calcium: 60mg

- Iron: 4mg

Instructions:

1. Heat olive oil in a large pot over medium heat. Add diced onion, carrots, and celery, and sauté until softened, about 5 minutes.

2. Add minced garlic and cook for another minute until fragrant.

3. Stir in rinsed lentils, vegetable broth, bay leaf, dried thyme, salt, and pepper.

4. Bring the soup to a boil, then reduce heat, cover, and simmer for 20-25 minutes, or until lentils are tender.

5. Remove bay leaf from the soup and discard.

6. Stir in chopped fresh parsley.

7. Ladle soup into bowls and serve hot with lemon wedges on the side.

8. Enjoy this hearty and nutritious lentil and vegetable soup for a comforting lunch option!

Mediterranean Chickpea Salad

Ingredients:

- 1 can (15 oz.) chickpeas, drained and rinsed

- 1 cucumber, diced

- 1 bell pepper, diced

- 1/2 red onion, finely chopped

- 1/4 cup chopped fresh parsley

- 1/4 cup crumbled feta cheese

- 2 tablespoons extra virgin olive oil

- 1 tablespoon red wine vinegar

- 1 teaspoon dried oregano

- Salt and pepper to taste

Prep Time: 10 mins

Total Time: 10 mins

Servings: 2

Nutrition Facts (per serving):

- Calories: 320

- Fat: 16g

- Saturated fat: 3g

- Cholesterol: 10mg

- Sodium: 380mg

- Carbohydrate: 36g

- Fiber: 10g

- Sugar: 7g

- Protein: 12g

- Vitamin C: 70mg

- Calcium: 140mg

- Iron: 4mg

Instructions:

1. In a large bowl, combine chickpeas, diced cucumber, diced bell pepper, chopped red onion, and chopped fresh parsley.

2. Add crumbled feta cheese to the bowl.

3. In a small bowl, whisk together extra virgin olive oil, red wine vinegar, dried oregano, salt, and pepper.

4. Pour the dressing over the chickpea salad and toss gently to coat evenly.

5. Serve Mediterranean chickpea salad immediately as a refreshing and nutritious lunch option!

Salmon and Avocado Salad

Ingredients:

- 2 salmon fillets

- 1 tablespoon olive oil

- Salt and pepper to taste

- 4 cups mixed salad greens

- 1 avocado, sliced

- 1/2 cup cherry tomatoes, halved

- 1/4 cup sliced red onion

- 2 tablespoons lemon juice

- 1 tablespoon balsamic vinegar

Prep Time: 10 mins

Cooking Time: 10 mins

Total Time: 20 mins

Servings: 2

Nutrition Facts (per serving):

- Calories: 350

- Fat: 22g

- Saturated fat: 3g

- Cholesterol: 60mg

- Sodium: 70mg

- Carbohydrate: 15g

- Fiber: 7g

- Sugar: 4g

- Protein: 25g

- Vitamin C: 20mg

- Calcium: 60mg

- Iron: 2mg

Instructions:

1. Preheat oven to 400°F (200°C).

2. Rub salmon fillets with olive oil and season with salt and pepper.

3. Place salmon fillets on a baking sheet lined with parchment paper and bake for 8-10 minutes, or until cooked through.

4. In a large bowl, toss mixed salad greens, sliced avocado, cherry tomatoes, and sliced red onion.

5. Divide the salad mixture between two plates.

6. Top each salad with a baked salmon fillet.

7. Drizzle lemon juice and balsamic vinegar over the salads.

8. Serve immediately and enjoy this delicious and nutritious salmon and avocado salad!

Turkey and Vegetable Stir-Fry

Ingredients:

- 2 tablespoons olive oil

- 2 cloves garlic, minced

- 1 teaspoon grated fresh ginger

- 2 cups mixed vegetables (such as bell peppers, broccoli, and snap peas), sliced

- 8 oz. turkey breast, thinly sliced

- 2 tablespoons reduced-sodium soy sauce

- 1 tablespoon honey or maple syrup (optional)

- Cooked brown rice or quinoa for serving

Prep Time: 10 mins

Cooking Time: 10 mins

Total Time: 20 mins

Servings: 2

Nutrition Facts (per serving):

- Calories: 320

- Fat: 12g

- Saturated fat: 2g

- Cholesterol: 50mg

- Sodium: 600mg

- Carbohydrate: 25g

- Fiber: 5g

- Sugar: 9g

- Protein: 30g

- Vitamin C: 70mg

- Calcium: 40mg

- Iron: 2mg

Instructions:

1. Heat olive oil in a large skillet or wok over medium-high heat.

2. Add minced garlic and grated ginger to the skillet and cook for 1 minute until fragrant.

3. Add sliced mixed vegetables to the skillet and stir-fry for 3-4 minutes until tender-crisp.

4. Push vegetables to one side of the skillet and add thinly sliced turkey breast to the other side. Cook until turkey is cooked through, about 3-4 minutes.

5. In a small bowl, whisk together reduced-sodium soy sauce and honey or maple syrup (if using). Pour over the stir-fry mixture.

6. Stir to combine all ingredients and cook for another 1-2 minutes.

7. Serve turkey and vegetable stir-fry hot over cooked brown rice or quinoa.

8. Enjoy this flavourful and nutrient-packed meal for lunch!

Tuna Salad Lettuce Wraps

Ingredients:

- 2 cans (5 oz. each) tuna, drained

- 1/4 cup plain Greek yogurt

- 1 tablespoon Dijon mustard

- 1 tablespoon lemon juice

- 1/4 cup diced celery

- 1/4 cup diced red onion

- Salt and pepper to taste

- 4 large lettuce leaves (such as butter or romaine)

Prep Time: 10 mins

__Total Time:__ 10 mins

__Servings:__ 2

__Nutrition Facts (per serving):__

- Calories: 180

- Fat: 4g

- Saturated fat: 0.5g

- Cholesterol: 45mg

- Sodium: 450mg

- Carbohydrate: 4g

- Fiber: 1g

- Sugar: 2g

- Protein: 30g

- Vitamin C: 6mg

- Calcium: 50mg

- Iron: 2mg

__Instructions:__

1. In a medium bowl, combine drained tuna, plain Greek yogurt, Dijon mustard, lemon juice, diced celery, and diced red onion.

2. Season with salt and pepper to taste and mix until well combined.

3. Lay out lettuce leaves on a clean work surface.

4. Divide tuna salad mixture evenly among the lettuce leaves.

5. Roll up the lettuce leaves to form wraps.

6. Serve tuna salad lettuce wraps immediately and enjoy this light and protein-rich lunch option!

Veggie and Hummus Wrap

Ingredients:

- 2 whole grain or spinach tortillas

- 1/2 cup hummus

- 1/2 cup shredded carrots

- 1/2 cup sliced cucumber

- 1/2 cup sliced bell peppers (any colour)

- 1/4 cup sliced red onion

- Handful of baby spinach leaves

Prep Time: 10 mins

Total Time: 10 mins

Servings: 2

Nutrition Facts (per serving):

- Calories: 250

- Fat: 8g

- Saturated fat: 1g

- Cholesterol: 0mg

- Sodium: 520mg

- Carbohydrate: 35g

- Fiber: 8g

- Sugar: 5g

- Protein: 10g

- Vitamin C: 40mg

- Calcium: 100mg

- Iron: 2mg

Instructions:

1. Lay out tortillas on a clean work surface.

2. Spread 1/4 cup of hummus evenly over each tortilla.

3. Layer shredded carrots, sliced cucumber, sliced bell peppers, red onion, and baby spinach leaves evenly over each tortilla.

4. Roll up the tortillas tightly to form wraps.

5. Slice each wrap in half diagonally.

6. Serve veggie and hummus wraps immediately and enjoy this fresh and satisfying lunch option!

Quinoa and Black Bean Salad

Ingredients:

- 1 cup cooked quinoa

- 1 can (15 oz.) black beans, drained and rinsed

- 1 cup cherry tomatoes, halved

- 1/2 cup diced red bell pepper

- 1/4 cup chopped fresh cilantro

- 2 tablespoons lime juice

- 1 tablespoon extra-virgin olive oil

- 1 teaspoon ground cumin

- Salt and pepper to taste

- Optional: Avocado slices for serving

Prep Time: 10 mins

Total Time: 10 mins

Servings: 2

Nutrition Facts (per serving):

- Calories: 280

- Fat: 6g

- Saturated fat: 1g

- Cholesterol: 0mg

- Sodium: 450mg

- Carbohydrate: 48g

- Fiber: 13g

- Sugar: 5g

- Protein: 13g

- Vitamin C: 60mg

- Calcium: 60mg

- Iron: 4mg

Instructions:

1. In a large bowl, combine cooked quinoa, black beans, cherry tomatoes, diced red bell pepper, and chopped fresh cilantro.

2. In a small bowl, whisk together lime juice, extra virgin olive oil, ground cumin, salt, and pepper.

3. Pour the dressing over the quinoa and black bean salad and toss gently to coat evenly.

4. Serve quinoa and black bean salad immediately, topped with avocado slices if desired.

5. Enjoy this protein-packed and flavourful salad for a satisfying lunch option!

Grilled Chicken and Vegetable Skewers

Ingredients:

- 2 boneless, skinless chicken breasts, cut into cubes
- 1 zucchini, sliced
- 1 yellow bell pepper, cut into chunks
- 1 red onion, cut into chunks
- 8 cherry tomatoes
- 2 tablespoons olive oil
- 2 cloves garlic, minced
- 1 teaspoon dried oregano
- Salt and pepper to taste

Prep Time: 15 mins

Cooking Time: 10 mins

Total Time: 25 mins

Servings: 2

Nutrition Facts (per serving):

- Calories: 320

- Fat: 12g

- Saturated fat: 2g

- Cholesterol: 90mg

- Sodium: 100mg

- Carbohydrate: 16g

- Fiber: 4g

- Sugar: 8g

- Protein: 35g

- Vitamin C: 90mg

- Calcium: 60mg

- Iron: 2mg

Instructions:

1. Preheat grill to medium-high heat.

2. In a bowl, combine olive oil, minced garlic, dried oregano, salt, and pepper.

3. Thread chicken cubes, sliced zucchini, bell pepper chunks, red onion chunks, and cherry tomatoes onto skewers.

4. Brush the skewers with the olive oil mixture.

5. Grill skewers for 8-10 minutes, turning occasionally, until chicken is cooked through and vegetables are tender.

6. Serve grilled chicken and vegetable skewers hot with a side of quinoa or brown rice, if desired.

Egg Salad Lettuce Wraps

Ingredients:

- 4 hard-boiled eggs, chopped

- 1/4 cup plain Greek yogurt

- 1 tablespoon Dijon mustard

- 2 tablespoons finely chopped celery

- 2 tablespoons finely chopped red onion

- Salt and pepper to taste

- 4 large lettuce leaves (such as butter or romaine)

Prep Time: 10 mins

Total Time: 10 mins

Servings: 2

Nutrition Facts (per serving):

- Calories: 160

- Fat: 10g

- Saturated fat: 2.5g

- Cholesterol: 370mg

- Sodium: 220mg

- Carbohydrate: 4g

- Fiber: 1g

- Sugar: 2g

- Protein: 13g

- Vitamin C: 2mg

- Calcium: 80mg

- Iron: 1mg

Instructions:

1. In a medium bowl, combine chopped hard-boiled eggs, plain Greek yogurt, Dijon mustard, chopped celery, and chopped red onion.

2. Season with salt and pepper to taste and mix until well combined.

3. Lay out lettuce leaves on a clean work surface.

4. Divide egg salad mixture evenly among the lettuce leaves.

5. Roll up the lettuce leaves to form wraps.

6. Serve egg salad lettuce wraps immediately for a light and protein-rich lunch.

Mediterranean Veggie Sandwich

Ingredients:

- 4 slices whole grain bread

- 1/4 cup hummus

- 1/2 cup sliced cucumber

- 1/2 cup sliced bell peppers (any colour)

- 1/4 cup sliced red onion

- 1/4 cup sliced Kalamata olives

- 1/4 cup crumbled feta cheese

- Handful of baby spinach leaves

Prep Time: 10 mins

Total Time: 10 mins

Servings: 2

Nutrition Facts (per serving):

- Calories: 280
- Fat: 10g
- Saturated fat: 3g
- Cholesterol: 15mg
- Sodium: 550mg
- Carbohydrate: 38g
- Fiber: 8g
- Sugar: 6g
- Protein: 11g
- Vitamin C: 30mg
- Calcium: 150mg
- Iron: 2mg

Instructions:

1. Toast the whole grain bread slices until lightly browned.
2. Spread 2 tablespoons of hummus on each slice of toasted bread.
3. Layer sliced cucumber, sliced bell peppers, sliced red onion, sliced Kalamata olives, crumbled feta cheese, and baby spinach leaves on two slices of bread.
4. Top with the remaining slices of bread to make sandwiches.
5. Slice sandwiches in half diagonally and serve immediately for a delicious and satisfying Mediterranean-inspired lunch.

Chickpea and Vegetable Curry

Ingredients:

- 1 tablespoon coconut oil

- 1 onion, diced

- 2 cloves garlic, minced

- 1 tablespoon grated fresh ginger

- 1 tablespoon curry powder

- 1 teaspoon ground turmeric

- 1 can (15 oz.) chickpeas, drained and rinsed

- 1 can (14 oz.) diced tomatoes

- 1 cup vegetable broth

- 2 cups chopped mixed vegetables (such as cauliflower, carrots, and bell peppers)

- Salt and pepper to taste

- Cooked brown rice for serving

Prep Time: 10 mins

Cooking Time: 20 mins

Total Time: 30 mins

Servings: 4

Nutrition Facts (per serving):

- Calories: 290

- Fat: 6g

- Saturated fat: 4g

- Cholesterol: 0mg

- Sodium: 680mg

- Carbohydrate: 49g

- Fiber: 13g

- Sugar: 10g

- Protein: 12g

- Vitamin C: 40mg

- Calcium: 100mg

- Iron: 4mg

Instructions:

1. In a large skillet, heat coconut oil over medium heat.

2. Add diced onion, minced garlic, and grated ginger to the skillet. Sauté until onion is soft and translucent, about 3-4 minutes.

3. Stir in curry powder and ground turmeric, and cook for another minute until fragrant.

4. Add drained and rinsed chickpeas, diced tomatoes, vegetable broth, and chopped mixed vegetables to the skillet. Season with salt and pepper to taste.

5. Bring the mixture to a simmer and cook for 15-20 minutes, stirring occasionally, until vegetables are tender and the curry has thickened.

6. Serve chickpea and vegetable curry hot over cooked brown rice for a hearty and flavourful lunch.

Caprese Salad with Balsamic Glaze

Ingredients:

- 2 large tomatoes, sliced

- 1 ball fresh mozzarella cheese, sliced

- Handful of fresh basil leaves

- 2 tablespoons balsamic glaze

- 1 tablespoon extra-virgin olive oil

- Salt and pepper to taste

Prep Time: 10 mins

Total Time: 10 mins

Servings: 2

Nutrition Facts (per serving):

- Calories: 220

- Fat: 15g

- Saturated fat: 6g

- Cholesterol: 30mg

- Sodium: 200mg

- Carbohydrate: 10g

- Fiber: 2g

- Sugar: 7g

- Protein: 10g

- Vitamin C: 20mg

- Calcium: 200mg

- Iron: 1mg

Instructions:

1. Arrange sliced tomatoes and sliced fresh mozzarella cheese on a serving platter.

2. Tuck fresh basil leaves in between the tomato and mozzarella slices.

3. Drizzle balsamic glaze and extra virgin olive oil over the salad.

4. Season with salt and pepper to taste.

5. Serve Caprese salad immediately as a light and refreshing lunch option.

DINNER RECIPES

Baked Salmon with Lemon and Dill

Ingredients:

- 4 salmon fillets

- 2 tablespoons olive oil

- 2 tablespoons freshly squeezed lemon juice

- 2 cloves garlic, minced

- 1 tablespoon chopped fresh dill

- Salt and pepper to taste

- Lemon wedges for serving

Prep Time: 10 mins

Cooking Time: 15 mins

Total Time: 25 mins

Servings: 4

Nutrition Facts (per serving):

- Calories: 280

- Fat: 15g

- Saturated fat: 2.5g

- Cholesterol: 80mg

- Sodium: 80mg

- Carbohydrate: 1g

- Fiber: 0g

- Sugar: 0g

- Protein: 32g

- Vitamin C: 8mg

- Calcium: 20mg

- Iron: 1mg

Instructions:

1. Preheat the oven to 400°F (200°C).

2. Place the salmon fillets on a baking sheet lined with parchment paper.

3. In a small bowl, whisk together olive oil, lemon juice, minced garlic, chopped dill, salt, and pepper.

4. Pour the lemon and dill mixture over the salmon fillets, ensuring they are evenly coated.

5. Bake in the preheated oven for 12-15 minutes, or until the salmon is cooked through and flakes easily with a fork.

6. Serve the baked salmon hot with lemon wedges on the side.

Quinoa Stuffed Bell Peppers

Ingredients:

- 4 bell peppers, halved and seeds removed

- 1 cup cooked quinoa

- 1 can (15 oz.) black beans, drained and rinsed

- 1 cup corn kernels (fresh or frozen)

- 1 cup diced tomatoes

- 1 teaspoon ground cumin

- 1 teaspoon chili powder

- Salt and pepper to taste

- 1/2 cup shredded cheddar cheese (optional)

- Fresh cilantro for garnish

Prep Time: 15 mins

Cooking Time: 30 mins

Total Time: 45 mins

Servings: 4

Nutrition Facts (per serving):

- Calories: 280

- Fat: 5g

- Saturated fat: 2g

- Cholesterol: 10mg

- Sodium: 350mg

- Carbohydrate: 48g

- Fiber: 11g

- Sugar: 8g

- Protein: 12g

- Vitamin C: 160mg

- Calcium: 120mg

- Iron: 4mg

Instructions:

1. Preheat the oven to 375°F (190°C).

2. In a large bowl, combine cooked quinoa, black beans, corn kernels, diced tomatoes, ground cumin, chili powder, salt, and pepper.

3. Stuff each bell pepper half with the quinoa mixture and place them in a baking dish.

4. Cover the baking dish with aluminium foil and bake in the preheated oven for 25 minutes.

5. Remove the foil, sprinkle shredded cheddar cheese (if using) over the stuffed bell peppers, and bake uncovered for an additional 5 minutes, or until the cheese is melted and bubbly.

6. Garnish with fresh cilantro before serving.

Turkey and Vegetable Stir-Fry

Ingredients:

- 1 tablespoon olive oil

- 1 lb turkey breast, thinly sliced

- 2 cups mixed vegetables (such as bell peppers, broccoli, and snap peas), sliced

- 3 cloves garlic, minced

- 1 tablespoon grated fresh ginger

- 1/4 cup reduced-sodium soy sauce

- 1 tablespoon honey or maple syrup (optional)

- Cooked brown rice for serving

Prep Time: 15 mins

Cooking Time: 15 mins

Total Time: 30 mins

Servings: 4

Nutrition Facts (per serving):

- Calories: 280

- Fat: 5g

- Saturated fat: 1g

- Cholesterol: 60mg

- Sodium: 600mg

- Carbohydrate: 25g

- Fiber: 5g

- Sugar: 9g

- Protein: 30g

- Vitamin C: 70mg

- Calcium: 40mg

- Iron: 2mg

Instructions:

1. Heat olive oil in a large skillet or wok over medium-high heat.

2. Add thinly sliced turkey breast to the skillet and cook until browned and cooked through, about 5-6 minutes. Remove from skillet and set aside.

3. In the same skillet, add minced garlic and grated ginger, and cook for 1 minute until fragrant.

4. Add sliced mixed vegetables to the skillet and stir-fry for 3-4 minutes until tender-crisp.

5. Push the vegetables to one side of the skillet and add the cooked turkey back to the skillet.

6. In a small bowl, whisk together reduced-sodium soy sauce and honey or maple syrup (if using). Pour over the stir-fry mixture.

7. Stir to combine all ingredients and cook for another 1-2 minutes.

8. Serve turkey and vegetable stir-fry hot over cooked brown rice.

Lentil and Vegetable Soup

Ingredients:

- 1 tablespoon olive oil

- 1 onion, diced

- 2 carrots, diced

- 2 celery stalks, diced

- 2 cloves garlic, minced

- 1 cup dried green lentils, rinsed

- 4 cups vegetable broth

- 1 bay leaf

- 1 teaspoon dried thyme

- Salt and pepper to taste

- 2 tablespoons chopped fresh parsley

- Lemon wedges for serving

Prep Time: 15 mins

Cooking Time: 30 mins

Total Time: 45 mins

Servings: 4

Nutrition Facts (per serving):

- Calories: 250

- Fat: 4g

- Saturated fat: 0.5g

- Cholesterol: 0mg

- Sodium: 580mg

- Carbohydrate: 38g

- Fiber: 15g

- Sugar: 6g

- Protein: 12g

- Vitamin C: 10mg

- Calcium: 60mg

- Iron: 4mg

Instructions:

1. Heat olive oil in a large pot over medium heat. Add diced onion, carrots, and celery, and sauté until softened, about 5 minutes.

2. Add minced garlic and cook for another minute until fragrant.

3. Stir in rinsed lentils, vegetable broth, bay leaf, dried thyme, salt, and pepper.

4. Bring the soup to a boil, then reduce heat, cover, and simmer for 20-25 minutes, or until lentils are tender.

5. Remove bay leaf from the soup and discard.

6. Stir in chopped fresh parsley.

7. Ladle soup into bowls and serve hot with lemon wedges on the side.

Mediterranean Chickpea Salad

Ingredients:

- 1 can (15 oz.) chickpeas, drained and rinsed

- 1 cucumber, diced

- 1 cup cherry tomatoes, halved

- 1/4 cup diced red onion

- 1/4 cup chopped fresh parsley

- 2 tablespoons extra virgin olive oil

- 1 tablespoon freshly squeezed lemon juice

- 1 teaspoon dried oregano

- Salt and pepper to taste

- Crumbled feta cheese for serving (optional)

Prep Time: 10 mins

Total Time: 10 mins

Servings: 4

Nutrition Facts (per serving):

- Calories: 180

- Fat: 8g

- Saturated fat: 1g

- Cholesterol: 0mg

- Sodium: 300mg

- Carbohydrate: 22g

- Fiber: 6g

- Sugar: 4g

- Protein: 7g

- Vitamin C: 20mg

- Calcium: 60mg

- Iron: 2mg

Instructions:

1. In a large bowl, combine drained and rinsed chickpeas, diced cucumber, halved cherry tomatoes, diced red onion, and chopped fresh parsley.

2. In a small bowl, whisk together extra virgin olive oil, lemon juice, dried oregano, salt, and pepper.

3. Pour the dressing over the chickpea salad and toss until well combined.

4. Serve Mediterranean chickpea salad cold or at room temperature.

5. Sprinkle crumbled feta cheese on top before serving, if desired.

Lemon Herb Grilled Chicken

Ingredients:

- 4 boneless, skinless chicken breasts

- 2 tablespoons olive oil

- Zest and juice of 1 lemon

- 2 cloves garlic, minced

- 1 tablespoon chopped fresh parsley

- 1 teaspoon chopped fresh thyme

- Salt and pepper to taste

Prep Time: 10 mins

Cooking Time: 15 mins

Total Time: 25 mins

Servings: 4

Nutrition Facts (per serving):

- Calories: 220

- Fat: 8g

- Saturated fat: 1.5g

- Cholesterol: 80mg

- Sodium: 90mg

- Carbohydrate: 1g

- Fiber: 0g

- Sugar: 0g

- Protein: 34g

- Vitamin C: 10mg

- Calcium: 20mg

- Iron: 1mg

1. In a bowl, whisk together olive oil, lemon zest, lemon juice, minced garlic, chopped parsley, chopped thyme, salt, and pepper.

2. Add chicken breasts to the bowl and toss to coat evenly with the marinade. Let marinate for at least 30 minutes, or up to 4 hours in the refrigerator.

3. Preheat grill to medium-high heat.

4. Remove chicken breasts from the marinade and discard excess marinade.

5. Grill chicken breasts for 6-7 minutes per side, or until cooked through and no longer pink in the centre.

6. Remove from grill and let rest for a few minutes before serving.

Vegetable Stir-Fry with Tofu

Ingredients:

- 1 tablespoon sesame oil

- 1 block (14 oz.) extra-firm tofu, pressed and cubed

- 2 cups mixed vegetables (such as bell peppers, broccoli, and snap peas), sliced

- 2 cloves garlic, minced

- 1 tablespoon grated fresh ginger

- 3 tablespoons reduced-sodium soy sauce

- 1 tablespoon rice vinegar

- 1 teaspoon honey or maple syrup (optional)

- Cooked brown rice for serving

Prep Time: 15 mins

Cooking Time: 15 mins

Total Time: 30 mins

Servings: 4

Nutrition Facts (per serving):

- Calories: 250

- Fat: 10g

- Saturated fat: 1.5g

- Cholesterol: 0mg

- Sodium: 400mg

- Carbohydrate: 20g

- Fiber: 4g

- Sugar: 5g

- Protein: 20g

- Vitamin C: 60mg

- Calcium: 200mg

- Iron: 3mg

Instructions:

1. Heat sesame oil in a large skillet or wok over medium-high heat.

2. Add cubed tofu to the skillet and cook until golden brown on all sides, about 5-6 minutes. Remove from skillet and set aside.

3. In the same skillet, add sliced mixed vegetables and stir-fry for 3-4 minutes until tender-crisp.

4. Push the vegetables to one side of the skillet and add minced garlic and grated ginger to the empty space. Cook for 1 minute until fragrant.

5. Return the cooked tofu to the skillet.

6. In a small bowl, whisk together reduced-sodium soy sauce, rice vinegar, and honey or maple syrup (if using). Pour over the stir-fry mixture.

7. Stir to combine all ingredients and cook for another 1-2 minutes.

8. Serve vegetable stir-fry with tofu hot over cooked brown rice.

Lemon Garlic Shrimp Pasta

Ingredients:

- 8 oz. whole grain spaghetti or pasta of choice

- 1 lb large shrimp, peeled and deveined

- 2 tablespoons olive oil

- 4 cloves garlic, minced

- Zest and juice of 1 lemon

- 1/4 teaspoon red pepper flakes

- Salt and pepper to taste

- 2 tablespoons chopped fresh parsley

Prep Time: 10 mins

Cooking Time: 10 mins

Total Time: 20 mins

Servings: 4

Nutrition Facts (per serving):

- Calories: 320

- Fat: 10g

- Saturated fat: 1.5g

- Cholesterol: 180mg

- Sodium: 140mg

- Carbohydrate: 35g

- Fiber: 6g

- Sugar: 2g

- Protein: 25g

- Vitamin C: 20mg

- Calcium: 60mg

- Iron: 3mg

Instructions:

1. Cook pasta according to package instructions until al dente. Drain and set aside.

2. Heat olive oil in a large skillet over medium heat.

3. Add minced garlic to the skillet and cook for 1 minute until fragrant.

4. Add shrimp to the skillet and cook for 2-3 minutes per side, until pink and cooked through.

5. Stir in lemon zest, lemon juice, red pepper flakes, salt, and pepper.

6. Add cooked pasta to the skillet and toss to coat evenly with the shrimp and lemon garlic sauce.

7. Cook for another 1-2 minutes, until heated through.

8. Sprinkle chopped fresh parsley over the pasta before serving.

Baked Cod with Herb Crust

Ingredients:

- 4 cod fillets

- 2 tablespoons olive oil

- 1/4 cup breadcrumbs (whole grain for added fiber)

- 1 tablespoon chopped fresh parsley

- 1 tablespoon chopped fresh dill

- 1 teaspoon chopped fresh thyme

- Zest of 1 lemon

- Salt and pepper to taste

- Lemon wedges for serving

Prep Time: 10 mins

Cooking Time: 15 mins

Total Time: 25 mins

Servings: 4

Nutrition Facts (per serving):

- Calories: 200

- Fat: 8g

- Saturated fat: 1.5g

- Cholesterol: 60mg

- Sodium: 200mg

- Carbohydrate: 5g

- Fiber: 1g

- Sugar: 0g

- Protein: 25g

- Vitamin C: 2mg

- Calcium: 20mg

- Iron: 1mg

Instructions:

1. Preheat the oven to 400°F (200°C). Line a baking sheet with parchment paper.

2. Place cod fillets on the prepared baking sheet.

3. In a small bowl, combine olive oil, breadcrumbs, chopped parsley, chopped dill, chopped thyme, lemon zest, salt, and pepper.

4. Spread the herb breadcrumb mixture evenly over the top of each cod fillet, pressing gently to adhere.

5. Bake in the preheated oven for 12-15 minutes, or until the cod is cooked through and flakes easily with a fork.

6. Remove from oven and let rest for a few minutes before serving.

7. Serve baked cod hot with lemon wedges on the side.

Vegetable and Tofu Coconut Curry

Ingredients:

- 1 tablespoon coconut oil

- 1 block (14 oz.) extra-firm tofu, pressed and cubed

- 1 onion, diced

- 2 cloves garlic, minced

- 1 tablespoon grated fresh ginger

- 2 tablespoons red curry paste

- 1 can (14 oz.) coconut milk

- 2 cups mixed vegetables (such as bell peppers, carrots, and snap peas)

- Salt and pepper to taste

- Cooked brown rice for serving

- Fresh cilantro for garnish

Prep Time: 15 mins

Cooking Time: 20 mins

Total Time: 35 mins

Servings: 4

Nutrition Facts (per serving):

- Calories: 350

- Fat: 25g

- Saturated fat: 20g

- Cholesterol: 0mg

- Sodium: 300mg

- Carbohydrate: 20g

- Fiber: 5g

- Sugar: 5g

- Protein: 15g

- Vitamin C: 30mg

- Calcium: 80mg

- Iron: 3mg

Instructions:

1. Heat coconut oil in a large skillet or pot over medium heat.

2. Add cubed tofu to the skillet and cook until golden brown on all sides, about 5-6 minutes. Remove from skillet and set aside.

3. In the same skillet, add diced onion, minced garlic, and grated ginger. Cook until onions are softened, about 3-4 minutes.

4. Stir in red curry paste and cook for another minute.

5. Pour in coconut milk and stir to combine with the curry paste mixture.

6. Add mixed vegetables to the skillet and simmer for 5-7 minutes, until vegetables are tender.

7. Return cooked tofu to the skillet and stir to coat evenly with the coconut curry sauce.

8. Season with salt and pepper to taste.

9. Serve vegetable and tofu coconut curry hot over cooked brown rice, garnished with fresh cilantro.

Turkey Meatballs with Zucchini Noodles

Ingredients:

- 1 lb lean ground turkey

- 1/4 cup breadcrumbs (whole grain for added fiber)

- 1 egg

- 2 cloves garlic, minced

- 1 teaspoon Italian seasoning

- Salt and pepper to taste

- 2 medium zucchinis, spiralized into noodles

- 1 cup marinara sauce (low-fat and low-sodium)

- Fresh basil leaves for garnish

Prep Time: 15 mins

Cooking Time: 20 mins

Total Time: 35 mins

Servings: 4

Nutrition Facts (per serving):

- Calories: 250

- Fat: 10g

- Saturated fat: 2g

- Cholesterol: 100mg

- Sodium: 300mg

- Carbohydrate: 10g

- Fiber: 3g

- Sugar: 5g

- Protein: 25g

- Vitamin C: 20mg

- Calcium: 60mg

- Iron: 3mg

Instructions:

1. Preheat oven to 400°F (200°C). Line a baking sheet with parchment paper.

2. In a large bowl, combine ground turkey, breadcrumbs, egg, minced garlic, Italian seasoning, salt, and pepper. Mix until well combined.

3. Roll mixture into golf ball-sized meatballs and place them on the prepared baking sheet.

4. Bake meatballs in the preheated oven for 15-20 minutes, or until cooked through and browned on the outside.

5. While the meatballs are baking, heat marinara sauce in a saucepan over medium heat.

6. Spiralize zucchinis into noodles using a spiralizer.

7. Once the meatballs are cooked, serve them over zucchini noodles and top with warm marinara sauce.

8. Garnish with fresh basil leaves before serving.

Baked Chicken and Vegetable Foil Packets

Ingredients:

- 4 boneless, skinless chicken breasts
- 2 cups mixed vegetables (such as bell peppers, zucchini, and carrots), diced
- 2 tablespoons olive oil
- 2 cloves garlic, minced
- 1 teaspoon Italian seasoning
- Salt and pepper to taste
- Lemon wedges for serving

Prep Time: 15 mins

Cooking Time: 25 mins

Total Time: 40 mins

Servings: 4

Nutrition Facts (per serving):

- Calories: 280

- Fat: 10g

- Saturated fat: 2g

- Cholesterol: 80mg

- Sodium: 150mg

- Carbohydrate: 10g

- Fiber: 3g

- Sugar: 4g

- Protein: 35g

- Vitamin C: 30mg

- Calcium: 40mg

- Iron: 2mg

Instructions:

1. Preheat oven to 400°F (200°C).

2. Cut four large squares of aluminium foil.

3. Place a chicken breast in the centre of each foil square.

4. In a bowl, toss diced mixed vegetables with olive oil, minced garlic, Italian seasoning, salt, and pepper.

5. Divide the vegetable mixture evenly among the foil packets, placing them around the chicken breasts.

6. Fold the sides of each foil packet over the chicken and vegetables to create a sealed packet.

7. Place the foil packets on a baking sheet and bake in the preheated oven for 20-25 minutes, or until the chicken is cooked through and vegetables are tender.

8. Carefully open the foil packets and serve the baked chicken and vegetable mixture hot with lemon wedges on the side.

Shrimp and Avocado Salad

Ingredients:

- 1 lb large shrimp, peeled and deveined

- 2 tablespoons olive oil

- 2 cloves garlic, minced

- 1 teaspoon paprika

- Salt and pepper to taste

- 4 cups mixed salad greens

- 1 avocado, diced

- 1 cup cherry tomatoes, halved

- 1/4 cup sliced red onion

- 2 tablespoons chopped fresh cilantro

- 2 tablespoons balsamic vinaigrette dressing (low-fat and low-sodium)

Prep Time: 15 mins

Cooking Time: 5 mins

Total Time: 20 mins

Servings: 4

Nutrition Facts (per serving):

- Calories: 280

- Fat: 15g

- Saturated fat: 2g

- Cholesterol: 200mg

- Sodium: 250mg

- Carbohydrate: 15g

- Fiber: 7g

- Sugar: 5g

- Protein: 25g

- Vitamin C: 30mg

- Calcium: 80mg

- Iron: 3mg

Instructions:

1. Heat olive oil in a large skillet over medium-high heat.

2. Add minced garlic and cook for 1 minute until fragrant.

3. Season peeled and deveined shrimp with paprika, salt, and pepper.

4. Add seasoned shrimp to the skillet and cook for 2-3 minutes per side, until pink and cooked through.

5. In a large bowl, toss mixed salad greens with diced avocado, halved cherry tomatoes, sliced red onion, and chopped fresh cilantro.

6. Divide the salad mixture among serving plates.

7. Top each salad with cooked shrimp.

8. Drizzle balsamic vinaigrette dressing over the shrimp and avocado salad before serving.

Veggie and Lentil Shepherd's Pie

Ingredients:

- 1 cup green lentils, rinsed

- 2 cups vegetable broth

- 2 tablespoons olive oil

- 1 onion, diced

- 2 carrots, diced

- 2 celery stalks, diced

- 2 cloves garlic, minced

- 1 cup frozen peas

- 1 teaspoon dried thyme

- Salt and pepper to taste

- 4 cups mashed potatoes (prepared without butter or cream)

Prep Time: 15 mins

Cooking Time: 40 mins

Total Time: 55 mins

Servings: 4

Nutrition Facts (per serving):

- Calories: 320

- Fat: 8g

- Saturated fat: 1g

- Cholesterol: 0mg

- Sodium: 600mg

- Carbohydrate: 50g

- Fiber: 12g

- Sugar: 7g

- Protein: 15g

- Vitamin C: 30mg

- Calcium: 60mg

- Iron: 4mg

Instructions:

1. Preheat oven to 375°F (190°C).

2. In a saucepan, combine rinsed green lentils and vegetable broth. Bring to a boil, then reduce heat and simmer for 20-25 minutes, or until lentils are tender and most of the liquid is absorbed. Drain any excess liquid and set aside.

3. In a large skillet, heat olive oil over medium heat. Add diced onion, carrots, and celery, and cook until softened, about 5-6 minutes.

4. Add minced garlic to the skillet and cook for 1 minute until fragrant.

5. Stir in cooked green lentils, frozen peas, dried thyme, salt, and pepper. Cook for another 2-3 minutes until heated through.

6. Transfer the lentil and vegetable mixture to a baking dish.

7. Spread mashed potatoes evenly over the top of the lentil mixture.

8. Bake in the preheated oven for 15-20 minutes, or until the mashed potatoes are lightly golden brown on top.

9. Remove from oven and let cool for a few minutes before serving.

Quinoa Stuffed Bell Peppers

Ingredients:

- 4 large bell peppers, halved and seeds removed

- 1 cup quinoa, rinsed

- 2 cups vegetable broth

- 1 tablespoon olive oil

- 1 onion, diced

- 2 cloves garlic, minced

- 1 zucchini, diced

- 1 cup canned black beans, drained and rinsed

- 1 cup corn kernels (fresh or frozen)

- 1 teaspoon ground cumin

- Salt and pepper to taste

- 1/4 cup chopped fresh cilantro

- 1/4 cup shredded cheddar cheese (optional)

Prep Time: 20 mins

Cooking Time: 30 mins

Total Time: 50 mins

Servings: 4

Nutrition Facts (per serving):

- Calories: 320

- Fat: 8g

- Saturated fat: 1.5g

- Cholesterol: 5mg

- Sodium: 450mg

- Carbohydrate: 55g

- Fiber: 12g

- Sugar: 8g

- Protein: 15g

- Vitamin C: 120mg

- Calcium: 120mg

- Iron: 4mg

Instructions:

1. Preheat oven to 375°F (190°C). Place halved bell peppers in a baking dish and set aside.

2. In a saucepan, combine rinsed quinoa and vegetable broth. Bring to a boil, then reduce heat and simmer for 15-20 minutes, or until quinoa is cooked and liquid is absorbed. Remove from heat and set aside.

3. In a large skillet, heat olive oil over medium heat. Add diced onion and cook until softened, about 5-6 minutes.

4. Add minced garlic to the skillet and cook for 1 minute until fragrant.

5. Stir in diced zucchini, black beans, corn kernels, ground cumin, salt, and pepper. Cook for another 5-6 minutes until vegetables are tender.

6. Add cooked quinoa to the skillet and stir to combine all ingredients.

7. Spoon quinoa mixture evenly into the halved bell peppers.

8. If using, sprinkle shredded cheddar cheese on top of each stuffed pepper.

9. Cover the baking dish with foil and bake in the preheated oven for 20-25 minutes, or until the peppers are tender.

10. Remove foil and bake for an additional 5 minutes to melt the cheese, if using.

11. Remove from oven and let cool for a few minutes before serving

APPETIZER RECIPES

Avocado and Tomato Bruschetta

Ingredients:

- 4 slices whole grain baguette

- 1 ripe avocado, mashed

- 1 medium tomato, diced

- 1 tablespoon chopped fresh basil

- 1 tablespoon balsamic vinegar

- Salt and pepper to taste

- Optional: extra virgin olive oil for drizzling

Prep Time: 10 mins

Cooking Time: 5 mins

Total Time: 15 mins

Servings: 2

Nutrition Facts (per serving):

- Calories: 160

- Fat: 8g

- Saturated fat: 1g

- Cholesterol: 0mg

- Sodium: 150mg

- Carbohydrate: 20g

- Fiber: 4g

- Sugar: 3g

- Protein: 4g

- Vitamin C: 10mg

- Calcium: 40mg

- Iron: 1mg

Instructions:

1. Preheat the oven to 375°F (190°C).

2. Place baguette slices on a baking sheet and toast in the oven for 5 minutes, or until lightly golden brown.

3. In a small bowl, combine mashed avocado, diced tomato, chopped basil, and balsamic vinegar. Season with salt and pepper to taste.

4. Remove toasted baguette slices from the oven and top each with a generous amount of the avocado and tomato mixture.

5. Optionally, drizzle with extra virgin olive oil before serving.

Cucumber and Hummus Bites

Ingredients:

- 1 English cucumber

- 1/2 cup hummus (store-bought or homemade)

- 1 tablespoon chopped fresh parsley

- Salt and pepper to taste

- Optional: paprika for garnish

Prep Time: 10 mins

Cooking Time: 0 mins

Total Time: 10 mins

Servings: 4

Nutrition Facts (per serving):

- Calories: 60

- Fat: 2.5g

- Saturated fat: 0g

- Cholesterol: 0mg

- Sodium: 150mg

- Carbohydrate: 8g

- Fiber: 2g

- Sugar: 1g

- Protein: 3g

- Vitamin C: 6mg

- Calcium: 20mg

- Iron: 1mg

Instructions:

1. Slice the cucumber into 1-inch-thick rounds.

2. Use a small spoon or a melon baller to scoop out a small portion of the centre of each cucumber round, creating a small well.

3. Fill each cucumber round with a dollop of hummus.

4. Sprinkle chopped parsley over the top of the hummus.

5. Season with salt and pepper to taste.

6. Optionally, garnish with a sprinkle of paprika before serving.

Spinach and Feta Stuffed Mushrooms

Ingredients:

- 12 large mushrooms, stems removed and reserved

- 2 cups fresh spinach, chopped

- 1/2 onion, finely chopped

- 2 cloves garlic, minced

- 1/4 cup crumbled feta cheese

- 1 tablespoon olive oil

- Salt and pepper to taste

Prep Time: 15 mins

Cooking Time: 20 mins

Total Time: 35 mins

Servings: 4

Nutrition Facts (per serving):

- Calories: 70

- Fat: 5g

- Saturated fat: 1.5g

- Cholesterol: 5mg

- Sodium: 100mg

- Carbohydrate: 5g

- Fiber: 1g

- Sugar: 2g

- Protein: 3g

- Vitamin C: 10mg

- Calcium: 50mg

- Iron: 1mg

Instructions:

1. Preheat the oven to 375°F (190°C).

2. Finely chop the mushroom stems.

3. Heat olive oil in a skillet over medium heat. Add chopped mushroom stems, onion, and garlic. Cook until softened, about 5 minutes.

4. Add chopped spinach to the skillet and cook until wilted, about 2-3 minutes.

5. Remove skillet from heat and stir in crumbled feta cheese. Season with salt and pepper to taste.

6. Place mushroom caps on a baking sheet, cavity side up.

7. Spoon the spinach and feta mixture into each mushroom cap.

8. Bake in the preheated oven for 15-20 minutes, or until mushrooms are tender and filling is heated through.

Caprese Skewers

Ingredients:

- 12 cherry tomatoes

- 12 small fresh mozzarella balls (bocconcini)

- 12 fresh basil leaves

- Balsamic glaze for drizzling

- Salt and pepper to taste

Prep Time: 10 mins

Cooking Time: 0 mins

Total Time: 10 mins

Servings: 4

Nutrition Facts (per serving):

- Calories: 90

- Fat: 6g

- Saturated fat: 3.5g

- Cholesterol: 20mg

- Sodium: 150mg

- Carbohydrate: 3g

- Fiber: 1g

- Sugar: 1g

- Protein: 6g

- Vitamin C: 10mg

- Calcium: 150mg

- Iron: 1mg

Instructions:

1. Thread one cherry tomato, one mozzarella ball, and one basil leaf onto each skewer.

2. Arrange skewers on a serving platter.

3. Drizzle with balsamic glaze.

4. Season with salt and pepper to taste.

5. Serve immediately.

Stuffed Bell Peppers with Creamy Avocado Dip

Ingredients:

- 2 large bell peppers, halved and seeds removed

- 1 avocado, peeled and pitted

- 1/4 cup Greek yogurt (low-fat and low-sodium)

- 1 tablespoon lime juice

- 1 clove garlic, minced

- 1/4 teaspoon ground cumin

- Salt and pepper to taste

- Optional: chopped fresh cilantro for garnish

Prep Time: 15 mins

Cooking Time: 0 mins

Total Time: 15 mins

Servings: 2

Nutrition Facts (per serving):

- Calories: 120

- Fat: 8g

- Saturated fat: 1.5g

- Cholesterol: 0mg

- Sodium: 20mg

- Carbohydrate: 12g

- Fiber: 6g

- Sugar: 3g

- Protein: 3g

- Vitamin C: 60mg

- Calcium: 20mg

- Iron: 1mg

Instructions:

1. In a blender or food processor, combine avocado, Greek yogurt, lime juice, minced garlic, ground cumin, salt, and pepper. Blend until smooth and creamy.

2. Spoon creamy avocado dip into each bell pepper half.

3. Optionally, garnish with chopped fresh cilantro before serving.

4. Serve immediately.

Greek Yogurt Veggie Dip

Ingredients:

- 1 cup Greek yogurt (low-fat and low-sodium)

- 1/2 cup finely chopped cucumber

- 1/4 cup finely chopped red bell pepper

- 1/4 cup finely chopped carrot

- 2 tablespoons finely chopped fresh dill

- 1 tablespoon lemon juice

- Salt and pepper to taste

- Assorted fresh vegetables for dipping (such as cucumber slices, carrot sticks, and bell pepper strips)

Prep Time: 10 mins

Cooking Time: 0 mins

Total Time: 10 mins

Servings: 4

Nutrition Facts (per serving):

- Calories: 60

- Fat: 1g

- Saturated fat: 0.5g

- Cholesterol: 5mg

- Sodium: 30mg

- Carbohydrate: 5g

- Fiber: 1g

- Sugar: 3g

- Protein: 8g

- Vitamin C: 20mg

- Calcium: 80mg

- Iron: 0.5mg

Instructions:

1. In a medium bowl, combine Greek yogurt, chopped cucumber, chopped red bell pepper, chopped carrot, chopped fresh dill, and lemon juice.

2. Stir until well combined.

3. Season with salt and pepper to taste.

4. Transfer the Greek yogurt veggie dip to a serving bowl.

5. Serve with assorted fresh vegetables for dipping.

Quinoa Salad Stuffed Endive Leaves

Ingredients:

- 1 cup cooked quinoa

- 1/4 cup diced cucumber

- 1/4 cup diced red bell pepper

- 2 tablespoons chopped fresh parsley

- 2 tablespoons lemon juice

- 1 tablespoon extra-virgin olive oil

- Salt and pepper to taste

- Endive leaves, separated

Prep Time: 15 mins

Cooking Time: 15 mins

Total Time: 30 mins

Servings: 4

Nutrition Facts (per serving):

- Calories: 80

- Fat: 3g

- Saturated fat: 0.5g

- Cholesterol: 0mg

- Sodium: 10mg

- Carbohydrate: 11g

- Fiber: 2g

- Sugar: 1g

- Protein: 2g

- Vitamin C: 10mg

- Calcium: 20mg

- Iron: 1mg

Instructions:

1. In a medium bowl, combine cooked quinoa, diced cucumber, diced red bell pepper, chopped fresh parsley, lemon juice, extra virgin olive oil, salt, and pepper.

2. Stir until well combined.

3. Spoon quinoa salad mixture into endive leaves, using each leaf as a boat.

4. Arrange stuffed endive leaves on a serving platter.

5. Serve immediately.

Smoked Salmon Cucumber Bites

Ingredients:

- 1 English cucumber

- 4 oz. smoked salmon, thinly sliced

- 1/4 cup Greek yogurt (low-fat and low-sodium)

- 1 tablespoon chopped fresh dill

- 1 teaspoon lemon zest

- Salt and pepper to taste

Prep Time: 15 mins

Cooking Time: 0 mins

Total Time: 15 mins

Servings: 4

Nutrition Facts (per serving):

- Calories: 70

- Fat: 3g

- Saturated fat: 1g

- Cholesterol: 10mg

- Sodium: 150mg

- Carbohydrate: 2g

- Fiber: 0g

- Sugar: 1g

- Protein: 10g

- Vitamin C: 10mg

- Calcium: 20mg

- Iron: 0.5mg

Instructions:

1. Cut the cucumber into thin rounds.

2. Place cucumber rounds on a serving platter.

3. Top each cucumber round with a slice of smoked salmon.

4. In a small bowl, combine Greek yogurt, chopped fresh dill, lemon zest, salt, and pepper.

5. Spoon a small dollop of the Greek yogurt mixture onto each smoked salmon-topped cucumber round.

6. Serve immediately.

Grilled Eggplant Rolls with Herbed Goat Cheese

Ingredients:

- 1 large eggplant, thinly sliced lengthwise

- 4 oz. goat cheese

- 1 tablespoon chopped fresh basil

- 1 tablespoon chopped fresh parsley

- 1 tablespoon chopped fresh chives

- 1 tablespoon extra-virgin olive oil

- Salt and pepper to taste

Prep Time: 20 mins

Cooking Time: 10 mins

Total Time: 30 mins

Servings: 4

Nutrition Facts (per serving):

- Calories: 120

- Fat: 8g

- Saturated fat: 4g

- Cholesterol: 15mg

- Sodium: 100mg

- Carbohydrate: 8g

- Fiber: 4g

- Sugar: 4g

- Protein: 6g

- Vitamin C: 8mg

- Calcium: 60mg

- Iron: 1mg

Instructions:

1. Preheat the grill or grill pan over medium-high heat.

2. Brush eggplant slices with olive oil and season with salt and pepper.

3. Grill eggplant slices for 2-3 minutes per side, or until tender and lightly charred. Remove from heat and let cool slightly.

4. In a small bowl, combine goat cheese, chopped fresh basil, chopped fresh parsley, and chopped fresh chives.

5. Spread a thin layer of the herbed goat cheese mixture onto each grilled eggplant slice.

6. Roll up the eggplant slices and secure with toothpicks, if necessary.

7. Arrange grilled eggplant rolls on a serving platter.

8. Serve warm or at room temperature.

Spinach and Artichoke Stuffed Mushrooms

Ingredients:

- 12 large mushrooms, stems removed and reserved

- 1 cup chopped fresh spinach

- 1/2 cup chopped canned artichoke hearts, drained

- 1/4 cup grated Parmesan cheese

- 1/4 cup Greek yogurt (low-fat and low-sodium)

- 2 cloves garlic, minced

- 1 tablespoon extra-virgin olive oil

- Salt and pepper to taste

Prep Time: 20 mins

Cooking Time: 20 mins

Total Time: 40 mins

Servings: 4

Nutrition Facts (per serving):

- Calories: 90

- Fat: 5g

- Saturated fat: 1.5g

- Cholesterol: 5mg

- Sodium: 150mg

- Carbohydrate: 7g

- Fiber: 2g

- Sugar: 2g

- Protein: 6g

- Vitamin C: 10mg

- Calcium: 80mg

- Iron: 1mg

Instructions:

1. Preheat the oven to 375°F (190°C).

2. Finely chop the mushroom stems.

3. In a skillet, heat olive oil over medium heat. Add chopped mushroom stems and minced garlic. Cook until softened, about 3-4 minutes.

4. Add chopped spinach and chopped artichoke hearts to the skillet. Cook until spinach is wilted and artichokes are heated through, about 2-3 minutes.

5. Remove skillet from heat and let cool slightly.

6. In a mixing bowl, combine cooked spinach and artichoke mixture, grated Parmesan cheese, and Greek yogurt. Stir until well combined. Season with salt and pepper to taste.

7. Spoon spinach and artichoke filling into each mushroom cap.

8. Place stuffed mushrooms on a baking sheet.

9. Bake in the preheated oven for 15-20 minutes, or until mushrooms are tender and filling is heated through.

Tomato Basil Bruschetta

Ingredients:

- 4 slices whole grain baguette

- 2 large tomatoes, diced

- 2 tablespoons chopped fresh basil

- 1 tablespoon extra-virgin olive oil

- 1 clove garlic, minced

- Salt and pepper to taste

Prep Time: 10 mins

Cooking Time: 5 mins

Total Time: 15 mins

Servings: 2

Nutrition Facts (per serving):

- Calories: 150

- Fat: 6g

- Saturated fat: 1g

- Cholesterol: 0mg

- Sodium: 150mg

- Carbohydrate: 20g

- Fiber: 4g

- Sugar: 4g

- Protein: 4g

- Vitamin C: 20mg

- Calcium: 40mg

- Iron: 1mg

Instructions:

1. Preheat the oven to 375°F (190°C).

2. Place baguette slices on a baking sheet and toast in the oven for 5 minutes, or until lightly golden brown.

3. In a bowl, combine diced tomatoes, chopped fresh basil, minced garlic, extra virgin olive oil, salt, and pepper.

4. Spoon tomato basil mixture onto toasted baguette slices.

5. Serve immediately.

Cucumber Avocado Sushi Rolls

Ingredients:

- 2 nori sheets

- 1/2 cup cooked sushi rice

- 1/2 avocado, sliced

- 1/2 cucumber, julienned

- Soy sauce for dipping (low-sodium)

- Pickled ginger and wasabi (optional)

Prep Time: 15 mins

Cooking Time: 0 mins

Total Time: 15 mins

Servings: 2

Nutrition Facts (per serving):

- Calories: 180

- Fat: 9g

- Saturated fat: 1.5g

- Cholesterol: 0mg

- Sodium: 150mg

- Carbohydrate: 22g

- Fiber: 5g

- Sugar: 1g

- Protein: 3g

- Vitamin C: 10mg

- Calcium: 10mg

- Iron: 1mg

Instructions:

1. Place a nori sheet on a sushi rolling mat or a clean kitchen towel.

2. Spread half of the sushi rice evenly over the nori sheet, leaving a small border along the edges.

3. Arrange avocado slices and cucumber julienne on top of the rice.

4. Carefully roll up the nori sheet, using the sushi rolling mat or kitchen towel to help shape the roll.

5. Repeat with the remaining nori sheet and ingredients.

6. Slice each sushi roll into 6-8 pieces.

7. Serve with soy sauce for dipping, and optionally, pickled ginger and wasabi.

Mediterranean Stuffed Cherry Tomatoes

Ingredients:

- 12 cherry tomatoes

- 1/4 cup crumbled feta cheese

- 2 tablespoons chopped Kalamata olives

- 1 tablespoon chopped fresh parsley

- 1 tablespoon extra-virgin olive oil

- Salt and pepper to taste

Prep Time: 15 mins

Cooking Time: 0 mins

Total Time: 15 mins

Servings: 2

Nutrition Facts (per serving):

- Calories: 90

- Fat: 7g

- Saturated fat: 2g

- Cholesterol: 10mg

- Sodium: 150mg

- Carbohydrate: 4g

- Fiber: 1g

- Sugar: 2g

- Protein: 3g

- Vitamin C: 20mg

- Calcium: 60mg

- Iron: 1mg

Instructions:

1. Cut the top off each cherry tomato and scoop out the seeds and pulp.

2. In a bowl, combine crumbled feta cheese, chopped Kalamata olives, chopped fresh parsley, and extra virgin olive oil. Season with salt and pepper to taste.

3. Stuff each cherry tomato with the feta cheese mixture.

4. Arrange stuffed cherry tomatoes on a serving platter.

5. Serve immediately or chill in the refrigerator until ready to serve.

Baked Sweet Potato Fries

Ingredients:

- 2 medium sweet potatoes, peeled and cut into fries

- 1 tablespoon corn-starch

- 1 tablespoon olive oil

- 1/2 teaspoon paprika

- 1/4 teaspoon garlic powder

- Salt and pepper to taste

Prep Time: 15 mins

Cooking Time: 25 mins

Total Time: 40 mins

Servings: 2

Nutrition Facts (per serving):

- Calories: 180

- Fat: 4g

- Saturated fat: 0.5g

- Cholesterol: 0mg

- Sodium: 150mg

- Carbohydrate: 34g

- Fiber: 5g

- Sugar: 7g

- Protein: 2g

- Vitamin C: 20mg

- Calcium: 40mg

- Iron: 1mg

Instructions:

1. Preheat the oven to 425°F (220°C).

2. In a large bowl, toss sweet potato fries with corn-starch, olive oil, paprika, garlic powder, salt, and pepper until evenly coated.

3. Spread sweet potato fries in a single layer on a baking sheet lined with parchment paper.

4. Bake in the preheated oven for 20-25 minutes, flipping halfway through, until fries are golden brown and crispy.

5. Remove from oven and let cool slightly before serving.

Caprese Salad Skewers

Ingredients:

- 12 cherry tomatoes

- 12 small fresh mozzarella balls (bocconcini)

- 12 fresh basil leaves

- Balsamic glaze for drizzling

- Salt and pepper to taste

Prep Time: 10 mins

Cooking Time: 0 mins

Total Time: 10 mins

Servings: 2

Nutrition Facts (per serving):

- Calories: 90

- Fat: 5g

- Saturated fat: 3g

- Cholesterol: 20mg

- Sodium: 150mg

- Carbohydrate: 4g

- Fiber: 1g

- Sugar: 2g

- Protein: 7g

- Vitamin C: 10mg

- Calcium: 150mg

- Iron: 1mg

Instructions:

1. Thread one cherry tomato, one mozzarella ball, and one basil leaf onto each skewer.

2. Arrange skewers on a serving platter.

3. Drizzle with balsamic glaze.

4. Season with salt and pepper to taste.

5. Serve immediately.

MAIN COURSE RECIPES

Grilled Lemon Herb Chicken

Ingredients:

- 4 boneless, skinless chicken breasts

- 2 tablespoons olive oil

- 2 tablespoons fresh lemon juice

- 2 cloves garlic, minced

- 1 teaspoon dried thyme

- 1 teaspoon dried rosemary

- Salt and pepper to taste

Prep Time: 10 mins

Marinating Time: 30 mins

Cooking Time: 12 mins

Total Time: 52 mins

Servings: 4

Nutrition Facts (per serving):

- Calories: 220

- Fat: 10g

- Saturated fat: 2g

- Cholesterol: 80mg

- Sodium: 280mg

- Carbohydrate: 1g

- Fiber: 0g

- Sugar: 0g

- Protein: 31g

- Vitamin C: 4mg

- Calcium: 20mg

- Iron: 1mg

Instructions:

1. In a bowl, whisk together olive oil, lemon juice, minced garlic, dried thyme, dried rosemary, salt, and pepper.

2. Place chicken breasts in a resalable plastic bag and pour the marinade over them. Seal the bag and refrigerate for at least 30 minutes.

3. Preheat grill to medium-high heat.

4. Remove chicken from marinade and discard excess marinade.

5. Grill chicken breasts for 6-7 minutes per side, or until cooked through and no longer pink in the centre.

6. Remove from grill and let rest for a few minutes before serving.

Baked Salmon with Dill Sauce

Ingredients:

- 4 salmon fillets

- 2 tablespoons olive oil

- 2 tablespoons lemon juice

- 2 cloves garlic, minced

- 2 tablespoons chopped fresh dill

- Salt and pepper to taste

Dill Sauce:

- 1/2 cup Greek yogurt (low-fat and low-sodium)

- 1 tablespoon chopped fresh dill

- 1 tablespoon lemon juice

- Salt and pepper to taste

Prep Time: 10 mins

Marinating Time: 30 mins

Cooking Time: 15 mins

Total Time: 55 mins

Servings: 4

Nutrition Facts (per serving):

- Calories: 280

- Fat: 15g

- Saturated fat: 3g

- Cholesterol: 80mg

- Sodium: 200mg

- Carbohydrate: 2g

- Fiber: 0g

- Sugar: 1g

- Protein: 33g

- Vitamin C: 4mg

- Calcium: 80mg

- Iron: 1mg

Instructions:

1. In a bowl, whisk together olive oil, lemon juice, minced garlic, chopped fresh dill, salt, and pepper.

2. Place salmon fillets in a resalable plastic bag and pour the marinade over them. Seal the bag and refrigerate for at least 30 minutes.

3. Preheat oven to 400°F (200°C).

4. Place marinated salmon fillets on a baking sheet lined with parchment paper.

5. Bake salmon for 12-15 minutes, or until fish flakes easily with a fork.

6. While salmon is baking, prepare the dill sauce by combining Greek yogurt, chopped fresh dill, lemon juice, salt, and pepper in a small bowl.

7. Serve baked salmon with dill sauce on the side.

Turkey and Vegetable Stir-Fry

Ingredients:

- 1 lb turkey breast, thinly sliced

- 2 tablespoons soy sauce (reduced-sodium)

- 1 tablespoon hoisin sauce

- 1 tablespoon corn-starch

- 2 tablespoons peanut or canola oil, divided

- 2 cups broccoli florets

- 1 red bell pepper, thinly sliced

- 1 yellow bell pepper, thinly sliced

- 1 carrot, julienned

- 2 cloves garlic, minced

- 1 teaspoon grated fresh ginger

- Cooked brown rice for serving

Prep Time: 15 mins

Cooking Time: 10 mins

Total Time: 25 mins

Servings: 4

Nutrition Facts (per serving):

- Calories: 280

- Fat: 10g

- Saturated fat: 1.5g

- Cholesterol: 60mg

- Sodium: 480mg

- Carbohydrate: 14g

- Fiber: 4g

- Sugar: 5g

- Protein: 30g

- Vitamin C: 120mg

- Calcium: 60mg

- Iron: 2mg

Instructions:

1. In a bowl, whisk together soy sauce, hoisin sauce, and corn-starch until smooth.

2. Add turkey slices to the bowl and toss to coat. Let marinate for 10 minutes.

3. Heat 1 tablespoon of oil in a wok or large skillet over high heat.

4. Add marinated turkey slices and stir-fry for 3-4 minutes, or until cooked through. Remove from wok and set aside.

5. Heat the remaining tablespoon of oil in the same wok or skillet.

6. Add broccoli florets, sliced red bell pepper, sliced yellow bell pepper, julienned carrot, minced garlic, and grated ginger. Stir-fry for 4-5 minutes, or until vegetables are tender-crisp.

7. Return cooked turkey slices to the wok and stir to combine with the vegetables.

8. Serve turkey and vegetable stir-fry over cooked brown rice.

Quinoa and Black Bean Salad

Ingredients:

- 1 cup quinoa, rinsed

- 2 cups water

- 1 can (15 oz.) black beans, drained and rinsed

- 1 cup cherry tomatoes, halved

- 1/2 cup chopped fresh cilantro

- 1/4 cup chopped red onion

- 1 avocado, diced

- 2 tablespoons extra virgin olive oil

- 2 tablespoons lime juice

- 1 teaspoon ground cumin

- Salt and pepper to taste

Prep Time: 10 mins

Cooking Time: 15 mins

Total Time: 25 mins

Servings: 4

Nutrition Facts (per serving):

- Calories: 320

- Fat: 15g

- Saturated fat: 2g

- Cholesterol: 0mg

- Sodium: 400mg

- Carbohydrate: 38g

- Fiber: 10g

- Sugar: 2g

- Protein: 10g

- Vitamin C: 15mg

- Calcium: 60mg

- Iron: 3mg

Instructions:

1. In a saucepan, bring water to a boil. Add quinoa, reduce heat to low, cover, and simmer for 12-15 minutes, or until water is absorbed and quinoa is cooked. Remove from heat and let cool.

2. In a large bowl, combine cooked quinoa, black beans, cherry tomatoes, chopped cilantro, chopped red onion, and diced avocado.

3. In a small bowl, whisk together extra virgin olive oil, lime juice, ground cumin, salt, and pepper.

4. Pour dressing over quinoa mixture and toss to coat evenly.

5. Serve quinoa and black bean salad chilled or at room temperature.

Vegetable and Tofu Stir-Fry

Ingredients:

- 1 block (14 oz.) extra firm tofu, pressed and cubed

- 2 tablespoons soy sauce (reduced-sodium)

- 1 tablespoon rice vinegar

- 1 tablespoon corn-starch

- 2 tablespoons peanut or canola oil, divided

- 2 cups broccoli florets

- 1 cup sliced mushrooms

- 1 red bell pepper, thinly sliced

- 1 yellow bell pepper, thinly sliced

- 2 cloves garlic, minced

- 1 teaspoon grated fresh ginger

- Cooked brown rice for serving

Prep Time: 20 mins

Cooking Time: 15 mins

Total Time: 35 mins

Servings: 4

Nutrition Facts (per serving):

- Calories: 240

- Fat: 12g

- Saturated fat: 1.5g

- Cholesterol: 0mg

- Sodium: 420mg

- Carbohydrate: 14g

- Fiber: 5g

- Sugar: 4g

- Protein: 20g

- Vitamin C: 130mg

- Calcium: 150mg

- Iron: 3mg

Instructions:

1. In a bowl, whisk together soy sauce, rice vinegar, and corn-starch until smooth.

2. Add cubed tofu to the bowl and toss to coat. Let marinate for 10 minutes.

3. Heat 1 tablespoon of oil in a wok or large skillet over high heat.

4. Add marinated tofu cubes and stir-fry for 4-5 minutes, or until golden brown. Remove from wok and set aside.

5. Heat the remaining tablespoon of oil in the same wok or skillet.

6. Add broccoli florets, sliced mushrooms, sliced red bell pepper, sliced yellow bell pepper, minced garlic, and grated ginger. Stir-fry for 4-5 minutes, or until vegetables are tender-crisp.

7. Return cooked tofu cubes to the wok and stir to combine with the vegetables.

8. Serve vegetable and tofu stir-fry over cooked brown rice.

Lemon Herb Grilled Shrimp Skewers

Ingredients:

- 1 lb large shrimp, peeled and deveined

- 2 tablespoons olive oil

- 2 tablespoons fresh lemon juice

- 2 cloves garlic, minced

- 1 tablespoon chopped fresh parsley

- 1 teaspoon dried oregano

- Salt and pepper to taste

Prep Time: 15 mins

Marinating Time: 30 mins

Cooking Time: 6 mins

Total Time: 51 mins

Servings: 4

Nutrition Facts (per serving):

- Calories: 180

- Fat: 10g

- Saturated fat: 1.5g

- Cholesterol: 160mg

- Sodium: 220mg

- Carbohydrate: 2g

- Fiber: 0g

- Sugar: 0g

- Protein: 20g

- Vitamin C: 10mg

- Calcium: 80mg

- Iron: 2mg

Instructions:

1. In a bowl, whisk together olive oil, lemon juice, minced garlic, chopped fresh parsley, dried oregano, salt, and pepper.

2. Add shrimp to the bowl and toss to coat. Let marinate for 30 minutes.

3. Preheat grill to medium-high heat.

4. Thread marinated shrimp onto skewers.

5. Grill shrimp skewers for 2-3 minutes per side, or until shrimp are opaque and cooked through.

6. Remove from grill and serve immediately.

Turkey and Vegetable Meatballs

Ingredients:

- 1 lb ground turkey

- 1/2 cup grated zucchini

- 1/2 cup grated carrot

- 1/4 cup finely chopped onion

- 2 cloves garlic, minced

- 1/4 cup chopped fresh parsley

- 1/4 cup grated Parmesan cheese

- 1 egg, beaten

- Salt and pepper to taste

- Marinara sauce for serving (low-sodium)

Prep Time: 15 mins

Cooking Time: 20 mins

Total Time: 35 mins

Servings: 4

Nutrition Facts (per serving):

- Calories: 220

- Fat: 10g

- Saturated fat: 3g

- Cholesterol: 120mg

- Sodium: 180mg

- Carbohydrate: 5g

- Fiber: 1g

- Sugar: 2g

- Protein: 25g

- Vitamin C: 10mg

- Calcium: 80mg

- Iron: 2mg

Instructions:

1. Preheat oven to 375°F (190°C). Line a baking sheet with parchment paper.

2. In a large bowl, combine ground turkey, grated zucchini, grated carrot, chopped onion, minced garlic, chopped parsley, grated Parmesan cheese, beaten egg, salt, and pepper. Mix until well combined.

3. Roll mixture into meatballs, about 1 inch in diameter, and place them on the prepared baking sheet.

4. Bake meatballs in the preheated oven for 18-20 minutes, or until cooked through and golden brown.

5. Serve turkey and vegetable meatballs with marinara sauce for dipping or over cooked pasta.

Lentil and Vegetable Curry

Ingredients:

- 1 cup dry green lentils, rinsed

- 2 cups water or vegetable broth

- 1 tablespoon olive oil

- 1 onion, diced

- 2 cloves garlic, minced

- 1 tablespoon grated fresh ginger

- 1 tablespoon curry powder

- 1 teaspoon ground cumin

- 1/2 teaspoon ground turmeric

- 1/4 teaspoon cayenne pepper (optional)

- 1 can (14 oz.) diced tomatoes

- 1 can (14 oz.) coconut milk

- 2 cups chopped vegetables (e.g., bell peppers, carrots, broccoli)

- Salt and pepper to taste

- Cooked brown rice or quinoa for serving

Prep Time: 10 mins

Cooking Time: 25 mins

Total Time: 35 mins

Servings: 4

Nutrition Facts (per serving):

- Calories: 320

- Fat: 15g

- Saturated fat: 10g

- Cholesterol: 0mg

- Sodium: 500mg

- Carbohydrate: 35g

- Fiber: 12g

- Sugar: 7g

- Protein: 12g

- Vitamin C: 30mg

- Calcium: 80mg

- Iron: 5mg

Instructions:

1. In a saucepan, bring water or vegetable broth to a boil. Add rinsed lentils, reduce heat to low, cover, and simmer for 15-20 minutes, or until lentils are tender. Drain any excess liquid and set aside.

2. In a large skillet, heat olive oil over medium heat. Add diced onion and cook until softened, about 5 minutes.

3. Add minced garlic, grated ginger, curry powder, ground cumin, ground turmeric, and cayenne pepper (if using) to the skillet. Cook for 1-2 minutes, or until fragrant.

4. Stir in diced tomatoes (with their juices) and coconut milk. Bring to a simmer.

5. Add chopped vegetables and cooked lentils to the skillet. Simmer for 5-7 minutes, or until vegetables are tender.

6. Season with salt and pepper to taste.

7. Serve lentil and vegetable curry over cooked brown rice or quinoa.

Baked Cod with Lemon and Herbs

Ingredients:

- 4 cod fillets

- 2 tablespoons olive oil

- 2 tablespoons fresh lemon juice

- 2 cloves garlic, minced

- 1 tablespoon chopped fresh parsley

- 1 tablespoon chopped fresh dill

- Salt and pepper to taste

- Lemon slices for garnish

Prep Time: 10 mins

Marinating Time: 30 mins

Cooking Time: 15 mins

Total Time: 55 mins

Servings: 4

Nutrition Facts (per serving):

- Calories: 200

- Fat: 8g

- Saturated fat: 1.5g

- Cholesterol: 70mg

- Sodium: 150mg

- Carbohydrate: 2g

- Fiber: 0g

- Sugar: 0g

- Protein: 30g

- Vitamin C: 4mg

- Calcium: 30mg

- Iron: 1mg

Instructions:

1. In a bowl, whisk together olive oil, lemon juice, minced garlic, chopped fresh parsley, chopped fresh dill, salt, and pepper.

2. Place cod fillets in a shallow dish and pour the marinade over them. Cover and refrigerate for 30 minutes.

3. Preheat oven to 400°F (200°C). Line a baking sheet with parchment paper.

4. Remove cod fillets from the marinade and place them on the prepared baking sheet.

5. Bake cod fillets in the preheated oven for 12-15 minutes, or until fish flakes easily with a fork.

6. Serve baked cod with lemon slices for garnish.

Vegetable and Chickpea Stew

Ingredients:

- 2 tablespoons olive oil

- 1 onion, diced

- 2 cloves garlic, minced

- 2 carrots, diced

- 2 celery stalks, diced

- 1 bell pepper, diced

- 1 zucchini, diced

- 1 can (14 oz.) diced tomatoes

- 1 can (14 oz.) chickpeas, drained and rinsed

- 2 cups vegetable broth

- 1 teaspoon dried oregano

- 1 teaspoon dried basil

- Salt and pepper to taste

- Chopped fresh parsley for garnish

Prep Time: 15 mins

Cooking Time: 25 mins

Total Time: 40 mins

Servings: 4

Nutrition Facts (per serving):

- Calories: 220

- Fat: 8g

- Saturated fat: 1g

- Cholesterol: 0mg

- Sodium: 400mg

- Carbohydrate: 30g

- Fiber: 8g

- Sugar: 8g

- Protein: 8g

- Vitamin C: 50mg

- Calcium: 80mg

- Iron: 3mg

Instructions:

1. In a large pot, heat olive oil over medium heat. Add diced onion and minced garlic, and cook until softened, about 5 minutes.

2. Add diced carrots, diced celery, diced bell pepper, and diced zucchini to the pot. Cook for another 5 minutes, or until vegetables start to soften.

3. Stir in diced tomatoes, drained and rinsed chickpeas, vegetable broth, dried oregano, dried basil, salt, and pepper.

4. Bring stew to a simmer, then reduce heat to low and cover. Let simmer for 15-20 minutes, or until vegetables are tender.

5. Taste and adjust seasoning if necessary.

6. Serve vegetable and chickpea stew hot, garnished with chopped fresh parsley.

Grilled Chicken Breast with Roasted Vegetables

Ingredients:

- 4 boneless, skinless chicken breasts

- 2 tablespoons olive oil

- 1 teaspoon garlic powder

- 1 teaspoon onion powder

- 1 teaspoon dried thyme

- 1 teaspoon dried rosemary

- Salt and pepper to taste

- 2 cups mixed vegetables (e.g., bell peppers, zucchini, cherry tomatoes)

- Cooking spray

Prep Time: 15 mins

Marinating Time: 30 mins

Cooking Time: 20 mins

Total Time: 65 mins

Servings: 4

Nutrition Facts (per serving):

- Calories: 250

- Fat: 10g

- Saturated fat: 2g

- Cholesterol: 90mg

- Sodium: 150mg

- Carbohydrate: 8g

- Fiber: 2g

- Sugar: 4g

- Protein: 30g

- Vitamin C: 40mg

- Calcium: 30mg

- Iron: 2mg

Instructions:

1. In a bowl, combine olive oil, garlic powder, onion powder, dried thyme, dried rosemary, salt, and pepper. Mix well.

2. Place chicken breasts in the bowl and coat them with the marinade. Let marinate in the refrigerator for 30 minutes.

3. Preheat grill to medium-high heat. Lightly grease the grill grates with cooking spray.

4. Place marinated chicken breasts on the grill and cook for 6-8 minutes per side, or until cooked through and no longer pink in the centre.

5. In the meantime, toss mixed vegetables with a drizzle of olive oil, salt, and pepper.

6. Place seasoned vegetables on a baking sheet and roast in the oven at 400°F (200°C) for 15-20 minutes, or until tender.

7. Serve grilled chicken breasts with roasted vegetables.

Quinoa Stuffed Bell Peppers

Ingredients:

- 4 large bell peppers (any colour), halved and seeds removed

- 1 cup quinoa, rinsed

- 2 cups vegetable broth

- 1 tablespoon olive oil

- 1 onion, diced

- 2 cloves garlic, minced

- 1 cup diced tomatoes

- 1 cup black beans, drained and rinsed

- 1 cup corn kernels

- 1 teaspoon chili powder

- 1 teaspoon ground cumin

- Salt and pepper to taste

- Chopped fresh cilantro for garnish

Prep Time: 15 mins

Cooking Time: 40 mins

Total Time: 55 mins

Servings: 4

Nutrition Facts (per serving):
- Calories: 300

- Fat: 6g

- Saturated fat: 1g

- Cholesterol: 0mg

- Sodium: 350mg

- Carbohydrate: 50g

- Fiber: 10g

- Sugar: 8g

- Protein: 12g

- Vitamin C: 100mg

- Calcium: 50mg

- Iron: 3mg

Instructions:

1. Preheat oven to 375°F (190°C). Arrange halved bell peppers in a baking dish.

2. In a saucepan, bring vegetable broth to a boil. Add rinsed quinoa, reduce heat to low, cover, and simmer for 15 minutes, or until quinoa is cooked and liquid is absorbed.

3. In a skillet, heat olive oil over medium heat. Add diced onion and minced garlic, and cook until softened, about 5 minutes.

4. Stir in diced tomatoes, black beans, corn kernels, chili powder, ground cumin, salt, and pepper. Cook for another 5 minutes, then add cooked quinoa to the skillet. Mix well.

5. Spoon quinoa mixture into each halved bell pepper until they are filled to the top.

6. Cover the baking dish with foil and bake in the preheated oven for 25-30 minutes, or until bell peppers are tender.

7. Garnish with chopped fresh cilantro before serving.

Salmon and Asparagus Foil Packets

Ingredients:

- 4 salmon fillets

- 2 bunches asparagus, trimmed

- 4 cloves garlic, minced

- 2 tablespoons olive oil

- 2 tablespoons lemon juice

- 1 teaspoon dried dill

- Salt and pepper to taste

- Lemon slices for garnish

Prep Time: 15 mins

Cooking Time: 20 mins

Total Time: 35 mins

Servings: 4

Nutrition Facts (per serving):

- Calories: 300

- Fat: 18g

- Saturated fat: 3g

- Cholesterol: 80mg

- Sodium: 150mg

- Carbohydrate: 8g

- Fiber: 4g

- Sugar: 2g

- Protein: 28g

- Vitamin C: 20mg

- Calcium: 80mg

- Iron: 4mg

Instructions:

1. Preheat oven to 400°F (200°C). Cut four large pieces of aluminium foil.

2. Place a salmon fillet in the centre of each piece of foil. Arrange asparagus spears around the salmon.

3. In a small bowl, whisk together minced garlic, olive oil, lemon juice, dried dill, salt, and pepper.

4. Drizzle the garlic-lemon mixture over the salmon and asparagus.

5. Fold the sides of the foil over the salmon and asparagus to create a packet, sealing tightly.

6. Place foil packets on a baking sheet and bake in the preheated oven for 15-20 minutes, or until salmon is cooked through and flakes easily with a fork.

7. Carefully open the foil packets and serve salmon and asparagus with lemon slices for garnish.

Turkey and Spinach Meatloaf

Ingredients:

- 1 lb ground turkey

- 1 cup chopped spinach

- 1/2 cup grated zucchini

- 1/2 cup grated carrot

- 1/4 cup diced onion

- 2 cloves garlic, minced

- 1/4 cup rolled oats

- 1/4 cup grated Parmesan cheese

- 1 egg, beaten

- 2 tablespoons tomato paste

- 1 tablespoon Worcestershire sauce

- 1 teaspoon dried thyme

- 1 teaspoon dried oregano

- Salt and pepper to taste

- Cooking spray

Prep Time: 15 mins

Cooking Time: 45 mins

Total Time: 60 mins

Servings: 4

Nutrition Facts (per serving):

- Calories: 250

- Fat: 10g

- Saturated fat: 2g

- Cholesterol: 100mg

- Sodium: 300mg

- Carbohydrate: 10g

- Fiber: 3g

- Sugar: 3g

- Protein: 30g

- Vitamin C: 10mg

- Calcium: 80mg

- Iron: 2mg

Instructions:

1. Preheat oven to 375°F (190°C). Lightly grease a loaf pan with cooking spray.

2. In a large bowl, combine ground turkey, chopped spinach, grated zucchini, grated carrot, diced onion, minced garlic, rolled oats, grated Parmesan cheese, beaten egg, tomato paste, Worcestershire sauce, dried thyme, dried oregano, salt, and pepper. Mix until well combined.

3. Transfer the turkey mixture to the prepared loaf pan and press it evenly into the pan.

4. Bake meatloaf in the preheated oven for 40-45 minutes, or until cooked through and browned on top.

5. Let meatloaf cool for a few minutes before slicing and serving.

Veggie Stir-Fry with Tofu

Ingredients:

- 1 block firm tofu, pressed and cubed

- 2 tablespoons soy sauce (reduced-sodium)

- 1 tablespoon rice vinegar

- 1 tablespoon sesame oil

- 1 tablespoon corn-starch

- 1 tablespoon olive oil

- 2 cloves garlic, minced

- 1 tablespoon grated fresh ginger

- 1 bell pepper, thinly sliced

- 1 cup broccoli florets

- 1 cup sliced mushrooms

- 1 cup snap peas

- 2 green onions, chopped

- Cooked brown rice for serving

Prep Time: 20 mins

Cooking Time: 15 mins

Total Time: 35 mins

Servings: 4

Nutrition Facts (per serving):

- Calories: 280

- Fat: 15g

- Saturated fat: 2g

- Cholesterol: 0mg

- Sodium: 450mg

- Carbohydrate: 20g

- Fiber: 6g

- Sugar: 4g

- Protein: 20g

- Vitamin C: 60mg

- Calcium: 250mg

- Iron: 4mg

Instructions:

1. In a bowl, combine cubed tofu, soy sauce, rice vinegar, sesame oil, and corn-starch. Toss until tofu is evenly coated. Let marinate for 10-15 minutes.

2. Heat olive oil in a large skillet or wok over medium-high heat. Add minced garlic and grated ginger, and cook until fragrant, about 1 minute.

3. Add marinated tofu to the skillet and cook until golden brown on all sides, about 5-7 minutes. Remove tofu from skillet and set aside.

4. In the same skillet, add bell pepper slices, broccoli florets, sliced mushrooms, and snap peas. Stir-fry for 3-4 minutes, or until vegetables are tender-crisp.

5. Return cooked tofu to the skillet and add chopped green onions. Stir to combine.

6. Serve veggie stir-fry with tofu over cooked brown rice.

SOUPS AND SALADS RECIPES

Quinoa and Vegetable Soup

Ingredients:

- 1 cup quinoa, rinsed

- 4 cups vegetable broth

- 1 tablespoon olive oil

- 1 onion, chopped

- 2 carrots, diced

- 2 celery stalks, diced

- 2 cloves garlic, minced

- 1 teaspoon dried thyme

- 1 teaspoon dried oregano

- Salt and pepper to taste

- Chopped fresh parsley for garnish

Prep Time: 10 mins

Cooking Time: 25 mins

Total Time: 35 mins

Servings: 4

Nutrition Facts (per serving):

- Calories: 200

- Fat: 4g

- Saturated fat: 0.5g

- Cholesterol: 0mg

- Sodium: 600mg

- Carbohydrate: 35g

- Fiber: 6g

- Sugar: 4g

- Protein: 7g

- Vitamin C: 10mg

- Calcium: 60mg

- Iron: 3mg

Instructions:

1. In a large pot, heat olive oil over medium heat. Add chopped onion, diced carrots, diced celery, and minced garlic. Cook until vegetables are softened, about 5 minutes.

2. Add rinsed quinoa to the pot and toast for 2 minutes, stirring occasionally.

3. Pour in vegetable broth and add dried thyme, dried oregano, salt, and pepper. Bring to a boil.

4. Reduce heat to low, cover, and simmer for 15-20 minutes, or until quinoa is cooked and vegetables are tender.

5. Taste and adjust seasoning if necessary.

6. Serve hot, garnished with chopped fresh parsley.

Spinach and Strawberry Salad

Ingredients:

- 4 cups baby spinach leaves

- 1 cup sliced strawberries

- 1/4 cup sliced almonds

- 1/4 cup crumbled feta cheese

- 2 tablespoons balsamic vinegar

- 1 tablespoon olive oil

- 1 teaspoon honey

- Salt and pepper to taste

Prep Time: 10 mins

Total Time: 10 mins

Servings: 4

Nutrition Facts (per serving):

- Calories: 120

- Fat: 7g

- Saturated fat: 2g

- Cholesterol: 5mg

- Sodium: 150mg

- Carbohydrate: 10g

- Fiber: 3g

- Sugar: 6g

- Protein: 4g

- Vitamin C: 30mg

- Calcium: 100mg

- Iron: 2mg

Instructions:

1. In a large salad bowl, combine baby spinach leaves, sliced strawberries, sliced almonds, and crumbled feta cheese.

2. In a small bowl, whisk together balsamic vinegar, olive oil, honey, salt, and pepper to make the dressing.

3. Drizzle the dressing over the salad and toss gently to coat.

4. Serve immediately as a refreshing salad option.

Lentil and Vegetable Soup

Ingredients:

- 1 cup dried lentils, rinsed

- 4 cups vegetable broth

- 1 tablespoon olive oil

- 1 onion, diced

- 2 carrots, diced

- 2 celery stalks, diced

- 2 cloves garlic, minced

- 1 teaspoon ground cumin

- 1 teaspoon paprika

- 1/2 teaspoon turmeric

- Salt and pepper to taste

- Chopped fresh cilantro for garnish

Prep Time: 10 mins

Cooking Time: 30 mins

Total Time: 40 mins

Servings: 4

Nutrition Facts (per serving):

- Calories: 220

- Fat: 4g

- Saturated fat: 0.5g

- Cholesterol: 0mg

- Sodium: 600mg

- Carbohydrate: 35g

- Fiber: 12g

- Sugar: 4g

- Protein: 12g

- Vitamin C: 10mg

- Calcium: 60mg

- Iron: 4mg

Instructions:

1. In a large pot, heat olive oil over medium heat. Add diced onion, diced carrots, diced celery, and minced garlic. Cook until vegetables are softened, about 5 minutes.

2. Add rinsed lentils to the pot and stir to combine with the vegetables.

3. Pour in vegetable broth and add ground cumin, paprika, turmeric, salt, and pepper. Bring to a boil.

4. Reduce heat to low, cover, and simmer for 20-25 minutes, or until lentils are tender.

5. Taste and adjust seasoning if necessary.

6. Serve hot, garnished with chopped fresh cilantro.

Greek Chickpea Salad

Ingredients:

- 2 cups cooked chickpeas (canned or cooked from dry)

- 1 cucumber, diced

- 1 bell pepper, diced

- 1/2 red onion, thinly sliced

- 1/4 cup chopped Kalamata olives

- 1/4 cup crumbled feta cheese

- 2 tablespoons lemon juice

- 2 tablespoons olive oil

- 1 teaspoon dried oregano

- Salt and pepper to taste

Prep Time: 15 mins

Total Time: 15 mins

Servings: 4

Nutrition Facts (per serving):

- Calories: 220

- Fat: 10g

- Saturated fat: 2g

- Cholesterol: 5mg

- Sodium: 300mg

- Carbohydrate: 25g

- Fiber: 7g

- Sugar: 5g

- Protein: 10g

- Vitamin C: 40mg

- Calcium: 100mg

- Iron: 3mg

Instructions:

1. In a large salad bowl, combine cooked chickpeas, diced cucumber, diced bell pepper, thinly sliced red onion, chopped Kalamata olives, and crumbled feta cheese.

2. In a small bowl, whisk together lemon juice, olive oil, dried oregano, salt, and pepper to make the dressing.

3. Drizzle the dressing over the salad and toss gently to coat.

4. Serve immediately as a satisfying and nutritious salad option.

Tomato Basil Soup

Ingredients:

- 2 tablespoons olive oil

- 1 onion, chopped

- 2 cloves garlic, minced

- 4 cups chopped tomatoes (fresh or canned)

- 2 cups vegetable broth

- 1/4 cup chopped fresh basil leaves

- Salt and pepper to taste

- Optional: 1/4 cup heavy cream or coconut milk for creaminess (omit for dairy-free)

Prep Time: 10 mins

Cooking Time: 25 mins

Total Time: 35 mins

Servings: 4

Nutrition Facts (per serving, without cream):

- Calories: 100

- Fat: 7g

- Saturated fat: 1g

- Cholesterol: 0mg

- Sodium: 600mg

- Carbohydrate: 10g

- Fiber: 3g

- Sugar: 6g

- Protein: 2g

- Vitamin C: 20mg

- Calcium: 60mg

- Iron: 2mg

Instructions:

1. In a large pot, heat olive oil over medium heat. Add chopped onion and minced garlic. Cook until softened and fragrant, about 5 minutes.

2. Add chopped tomatoes to the pot and cook for 5 minutes, stirring occasionally.

3. Pour in vegetable broth and bring to a simmer. Cook for 15 minutes, allowing flavors to meld.

4. Remove the soup from heat and use an immersion blender to puree until smooth. Alternatively, transfer the soup to a blender and blend until smooth, then return to the pot.

5. Stir in chopped fresh basil leaves and season with salt and pepper to taste.

6. If using, stir in heavy cream or coconut milk for added creaminess.

7. Serve hot, garnished with additional fresh basil leaves if desired.

Lentil and Kale Soup

Ingredients:

- 1 cup dried green lentils, rinsed

- 4 cups vegetable broth

- 1 tablespoon olive oil

- 1 onion, chopped

- 2 carrots, diced

- 2 celery stalks, diced

- 2 cloves garlic, minced

- 2 cups chopped kale leaves

- 1 teaspoon ground cumin

- 1 teaspoon ground turmeric

- Salt and pepper to taste

- Lemon wedges for serving

Prep Time: 10 mins

Cooking Time: 30 mins

Total Time: 40 mins

Servings: 4

Nutrition Facts (per serving):

- Calories: 220

- Fat: 4g

- Saturated fat: 0.5g

- Cholesterol: 0mg

- Sodium: 600mg

- Carbohydrate: 35g

- Fiber: 12g

- Sugar: 4g

- Protein: 12g

- Vitamin C: 40mg

- Calcium: 100mg

- Iron: 4mg

Instructions:

1. In a large pot, heat olive oil over medium heat. Add chopped onion, diced carrots, diced celery, and minced garlic. Cook until vegetables are softened, about 5 minutes.

2. Add rinsed lentils to the pot and stir to combine with the vegetables.

3. Pour in vegetable broth and bring to a boil.

4. Reduce heat to low, cover, and simmer for 20-25 minutes, or until lentils are tender.

5. Stir in chopped kale leaves and cook for an additional 5 minutes, until kale is wilted.

6. Season with ground cumin, ground turmeric, salt, and pepper to taste.

7. Serve hot with lemon wedges for squeezing over the soup.

Greek Quinoa Salad

Ingredients:

- 1 cup cooked quinoa

- 1 cucumber, diced

- 1 bell pepper, diced

- 1/2 red onion, thinly sliced

- 1/4 cup pitted Kalamata olives, halved

- 1/4 cup crumbled feta cheese

- 2 tablespoons olive oil

- 2 tablespoons red wine vinegar

- 1 teaspoon dried oregano

- Salt and pepper to taste

Prep Time: 15 mins

Total Time: 15 mins

Servings: 4

Nutrition Facts (per serving):

- Calories: 220

- Fat: 10g

- Saturated fat: 2g

- Cholesterol: 5mg

- Sodium: 300mg

- Carbohydrate: 25g

- Fiber: 7g

- Sugar: 5g

- Protein: 10g

- Vitamin C: 40mg

- Calcium: 100mg

- Iron: 3mg

Instructions:

1. In a large salad bowl, combine cooked quinoa, diced cucumber, diced bell pepper, thinly sliced red onion, halved Kalamata olives, and crumbled feta cheese.

2. In a small bowl, whisk together olive oil, red wine vinegar, dried oregano, salt, and pepper to make the dressing.

3. Drizzle the dressing over the salad and toss gently to coat.

4. Serve immediately as a refreshing salad option.

Butternut Squash Soup

Ingredients:

- 1 butternut squash, peeled, seeded, and diced

- 1 onion, chopped

- 2 carrots, diced

- 2 celery stalks, diced

- 2 cloves garlic, minced

- 4 cups vegetable broth

- 1 teaspoon ground cinnamon

- 1/2 teaspoon ground nutmeg

- Salt and pepper to taste

- Optional: Greek yogurt or coconut cream for garnish

Prep Time: 15 mins

Cooking Time: 30 mins

Total Time: 45 mins

Servings: 4

Nutrition Facts (per serving):

- Calories: 150

- Fat: 1g

- Saturated fat: 0.5g

- Cholesterol: 0mg

- Sodium: 600mg

- Carbohydrate: 35g

- Fiber: 8g

- Sugar: 8g

- Protein: 4g

- Vitamin C: 50mg

- Calcium: 100mg

- Iron: 2mg

Instructions:

1. In a large pot, combine diced butternut squash, chopped onion, diced carrots, diced celery, minced garlic, and vegetable broth.

2. Bring the mixture to a boil, then reduce heat to low and simmer for 20-25 minutes, or until vegetables are tender.

3. Use an immersion blender to puree the soup until smooth. Alternatively, transfer the soup to a blender and blend until smooth, then return to the pot.

4. Stir in ground cinnamon, ground nutmeg, salt, and pepper to taste.

5. Serve hot, garnished with a dollop of Greek yogurt or coconut cream if desired.

Mediterranean Chickpea Salad

Ingredients:

- 2 cups cooked chickpeas (canned or cooked from dry)

- 1 cup diced cucumber

- 1 cup cherry tomatoes, halved

- 1/4 cup sliced red onion

- 1/4 cup chopped fresh parsley

- 2 tablespoons lemon juice

- 2 tablespoons extra virgin olive oil

- 1 teaspoon dried oregano

- Salt and pepper to taste

Prep Time: 15 mins

Total Time: 15 mins

Servings: 4

Nutrition Facts (per serving):

- Calories: 220

- Fat: 10g

- Saturated fat: 2g

- Cholesterol: 0mg

- Sodium: 300mg

- Carbohydrate: 25g

- Fiber: 8g

- Sugar: 5g

- Protein: 10g

- Vitamin C: 30mg

- Calcium: 100mg

- Iron: 3mg

Instructions:

1. In a large salad bowl, combine cooked chickpeas, diced cucumber, halved cherry tomatoes, sliced red onion, and chopped fresh parsley.

2. In a small bowl, whisk together lemon juice, extra virgin olive oil, dried oregano, salt, and pepper to make the dressing.

3. Drizzle the dressing over the salad and toss gently to coat.

4. Serve immediately as a flavourful and nutritious salad option.

Creamy Cauliflower Soup

Ingredients:

- 1 medium cauliflower head, chopped into florets

- 1 onion, chopped

- 2 cloves garlic, minced

- 4 cups vegetable broth

- 1/2 cup unsweetened almond milk or coconut milk

- Salt and pepper to taste

- Chopped fresh chives for garnish

Prep Time: 10 mins

Cooking Time: 25 mins

Total Time: 35 mins

Servings: 4

Nutrition Facts (per serving):

- Calories: 100

- Fat: 3g

- Saturated fat: 0.5g

- Cholesterol: 0mg

- Sodium: 600mg

- Carbohydrate: 15g

- Fiber: 6g

- Sugar: 6g

- Protein: 4g

- Vitamin C: 70mg

- Calcium: 100mg

- Iron: 2mg

Instructions:

1. In a large pot, combine chopped cauliflower florets, chopped onion, minced garlic, and vegetable broth.

2. Bring the mixture to a boil, then reduce heat to low and simmer for 20-25 minutes, or until cauliflower is tender.

3. Use an immersion blender to puree the soup until smooth. Alternatively, transfer the soup to a blender and blend until smooth, then return to the pot.

4. Stir in unsweetened almond milk or coconut milk to add creaminess.

5. Season with salt and pepper to taste.

6. Serve hot, garnished with chopped fresh chives for added flavor.

Spinach and Quinoa Salad

Ingredients:

- 1 cup cooked quinoa

- 2 cups fresh spinach leaves

- 1 cup cherry tomatoes, halved

- 1/4 cup sliced red onion

- 1/4 cup crumbled feta cheese

- 2 tablespoons olive oil

- 1 tablespoon balsamic vinegar

- 1 teaspoon Dijon mustard

- Salt and pepper to taste

Prep Time: 15 mins

Total Time: 15 mins

Servings: 4

Nutrition Facts (per serving):

- Calories: 180

- Fat: 8g

- Saturated fat: 2g

- Cholesterol: 5mg

- Sodium: 200mg

- Carbohydrate: 20g

- Fiber: 4g

- Sugar: 2g

- Protein: 6g

- Vitamin C: 20mg

- Calcium: 100mg

- Iron: 3mg

Instructions:

1. In a large salad bowl, combine cooked quinoa, fresh spinach leaves, halved cherry tomatoes, sliced red onion, and crumbled feta cheese.

2. In a small bowl, whisk together olive oil, balsamic vinegar, Dijon mustard, salt, and pepper to make the dressing.

3. Drizzle the dressing over the salad and toss gently to coat.

4. Serve immediately as a nutritious and satisfying salad option.

Carrot Ginger Soup

Ingredients:

- 1 tablespoon olive oil

- 1 onion, chopped

- 2 cloves garlic, minced

- 1 tablespoon grated fresh ginger

- 4 cups chopped carrots

- 4 cups vegetable broth

- Salt and pepper to taste

- Fresh cilantro leaves for garnish

Prep Time: 10 mins

Cooking Time: 25 mins

Total Time: 35 mins

Servings: 4

Nutrition Facts (per serving):

- Calories: 120

- Fat: 4g

- Saturated fat: 0.5g

- Cholesterol: 0mg

- Sodium: 600mg

- Carbohydrate: 20g

- Fiber: 6g

- Sugar: 8g

- Protein: 2g

- Vitamin C: 20mg

- Calcium: 80mg

- Iron: 1mg

Instructions:

1. In a large pot, heat olive oil over medium heat. Add chopped onion and minced garlic. Cook until softened and fragrant, about 5 minutes.

2. Add grated fresh ginger and chopped carrots to the pot. Cook for another 5 minutes, stirring occasionally.

3. Pour in vegetable broth and bring to a boil. Reduce heat to low, cover, and simmer for 15-20 minutes, or until carrots are tender.

4. Use an immersion blender to puree the soup until smooth. Alternatively, transfer the soup to a blender and blend until smooth, then return to the pot.

5. Season with salt and pepper to taste.

6. Serve hot, garnished with fresh cilantro leaves for added flavor.

Avocado and Tomato Salad

Ingredients:

- 2 ripe avocados, diced

- 2 cups cherry tomatoes, halved

- 1/4 cup chopped fresh cilantro

- 1/4 cup chopped red onion

- 2 tablespoons lime juice

- 1 tablespoon extra-virgin olive oil

- Salt and pepper to taste

Prep Time: 10 mins

Total Time: 10 mins

Servings: 4

Nutrition Facts (per serving):

- Calories: 180

- Fat: 15g

- Saturated fat: 2g

- Cholesterol: 0mg

- Sodium: 10mg

- Carbohydrate: 15g

- Fiber: 7g

- Sugar: 2g

- Protein: 3g

- Vitamin C: 20mg

- Calcium: 20mg

- Iron: 1mg

Instructions:

1. In a large salad bowl, combine diced avocados, halved cherry tomatoes, chopped fresh cilantro, and chopped red onion.

2. In a small bowl, whisk together lime juice, extra virgin olive oil, salt, and pepper to make the dressing.

3. Drizzle the dressing over the salad and toss gently to coat.

4. Serve immediately as a refreshing and nutritious salad option.

Potato Leek Soup

Ingredients:

- 2 tablespoons unsalted butter

- 2 leeks, white and light green parts only, thinly sliced

- 2 cloves garlic, minced

- 4 cups diced potatoes

- 4 cups vegetable broth

- 1/2 cup unsweetened almond milk or coconut milk

- Salt and pepper to taste

- Chopped fresh chives for garnish

Prep Time: 10 mins

Cooking Time: 25 mins

Total Time: 35 mins

Servings: 4

Nutrition Facts (per serving):

- Calories: 200

- Fat: 6g

- Saturated fat: 3g

- Cholesterol: 10mg

- Sodium: 500mg

- Carbohydrate: 30g

- Fiber: 4g

- Sugar: 4g

- Protein: 4g

- Vitamin C: 30mg

- Calcium: 40mg

- Iron: 2mg

Instructions:

1. In a large pot, melt unsalted butter over medium heat. Add thinly sliced leeks and minced garlic. Cook until softened and fragrant, about 5 minutes.

2. Add diced potatoes to the pot and stir to combine with the leeks and garlic.

3. Pour in vegetable broth and bring to a boil. Reduce heat to low, cover, and simmer for 15-20 minutes, or until potatoes are tender.

4. Use an immersion blender to puree the soup until smooth. Alternatively, transfer the soup to a blender and blend until smooth, then return to the pot.

5. Stir in unsweetened almond milk or coconut milk to add creaminess.

6. Season with salt and pepper to taste.

7. Serve hot, garnished with chopped fresh chives for added flavor.

Chickpea and Tomato Salad

Ingredients:

- 2 cups cooked chickpeas (canned or cooked from dry)

- 2 cups cherry tomatoes, halved

- 1/4 cup chopped fresh basil

- 1/4 cup crumbled feta cheese

- 2 tablespoons extra virgin olive oil

- 1 tablespoon balsamic vinegar

- Salt and pepper to taste

Prep Time: 10 mins

Total Time: 10 mins

Servings: 4

Nutrition Facts (per serving):

- Calories: 220

- Fat: 10g

- Saturated fat: 2g

- Cholesterol: 5mg

- Sodium: 300mg

- Carbohydrate: 25g

- Fiber: 7g

- Sugar: 5g

- Protein: 10g

- Vitamin C: 30mg

- Calcium: 100mg

- Iron: 3mg

Instructions:

1. In a large salad bowl, combine cooked chickpeas, halved cherry tomatoes, chopped fresh basil, and crumbled feta cheese.

2. In a small bowl, whisk together extra virgin olive oil, balsamic vinegar, salt, and pepper to make the dressing.

3. Drizzle the dressing over the salad and toss gently to coat.

4. Serve immediately as a satisfying and flavourful salad option.

14 DAY MEAL PLAN

Day 1:

- *Breakfast:* Almond Butter Banana Bites

- *Lunch:* Greek Yogurt Parfait

- *Dinner:* Baked Pears with Cinnamon and Honey

Day 2:

- *Breakfast:* Coconut Flour Pancakes

- *Lunch:* Chocolate Avocado Mousse

- *Dinner:* Pineapple Coconut Sorbet

Day 3:

- *Breakfast:* Almond Butter Banana Bites

- *Lunch:* Greek Yogurt Parfait

- *Dinner:* Baked Pears with Cinnamon and Honey

Day 4:

- *Breakfast:* Coconut Flour Pancakes

- *Lunch:* Chocolate Avocado Mousse

- *Dinner:* Pineapple Coconut Sorbet

Day 5:

- *Breakfast:* Almond Butter Banana Bites

- *Lunch:* Greek Yogurt Parfait

- *Dinner:* Baked Pears with Cinnamon and Honey

Day 6:

- *Breakfast:* Coconut Flour Pancakes

- *Lunch:* Chocolate Avocado Mousse

- *Dinner:* Pineapple Coconut Sorbet

Day 7:

- *Breakfast:* Almond Butter Banana Bites

- *Lunch:* Greek Yogurt Parfait

- *Dinner:* Baked Pears with Cinnamon and Honey

Day 8:

- *Breakfast:* Coconut Flour Pancakes

- *Lunch:* Almond Butter Banana Bites

- *Dinner:* Greek Yogurt Parfait

Day 9:

- *Breakfast:* Chocolate Avocado Mousse

- *Lunch:* Pineapple Coconut Sorbet

- *Dinner:* Baked Pears with Cinnamon and Honey

Day 10:

- *Breakfast:* Almond Butter Banana Bites

- *Lunch:* Coconut Flour Pancakes

- *Dinner:* Greek Yogurt Parfait

Day 11:

- *Breakfast:* Chocolate Avocado Mousse

- *Lunch:* Pineapple Coconut Sorbet

- *Dinner:* Baked Pears with Cinnamon and Honey

Day 12:

- *Breakfast:* Almond Butter Banana Bites

- *Lunch:* Coconut Flour Pancakes

- *Dinner:* Greek Yogurt Parfait

Day 13:

- *Breakfast:* Chocolate Avocado Mousse

- *Lunch:* Pineapple Coconut Sorbet

- *Dinner:* Baked Pears with Cinnamon and Honey

Day 14:

- *Breakfast:* Almond Butter Banana Bites

- *Lunch:* Coconut Flour Pancakes

- *Dinner:* Greek Yogurt Parfait

CONCLUSION

In conclusion, designing a meal plan for individuals with Exocrine Pancreatic Insufficiency (EPI) requires careful consideration of dietary restrictions and nutritional needs. Throughout our discussion, we've explored various recipes tailored to support individuals managing EPI, focusing on lean proteins, healthy fats, low-FODMAP carbohydrates, fibre-rich foods, and mindful dessert options.

By understanding the fundamentals of EPI, including its causes, symptoms, and diagnosis, as well as the importance of digestive enzymes and key nutrients, individuals can make informed dietary choices to support their overall health and well-being. Additionally, we've highlighted the significance of stress management techniques, regular exercise, and proper hydration in complementing a balanced diet for individuals with EPI.

Our meal plans offer a diverse range of flavourful and nutritious options, from breakfast to dessert, ensuring that individuals with EPI can enjoy delicious meals while adhering to their dietary requirements. Whether it's starting the day with coconut flour pancakes or winding down with baked pears and cinnamon, these recipes provide both nourishment and satisfaction.

Ultimately, by embracing a holistic approach to nutrition and lifestyle management, individuals with EPI can optimize their health outcomes and enhance their quality of life. With a focus on wholesome ingredients, mindful eating practices, and delicious meal options, navigating an EPI diet meal plan becomes not only manageable but also enjoyable. Here's to embracing a healthy and delicious journey towards wellness!

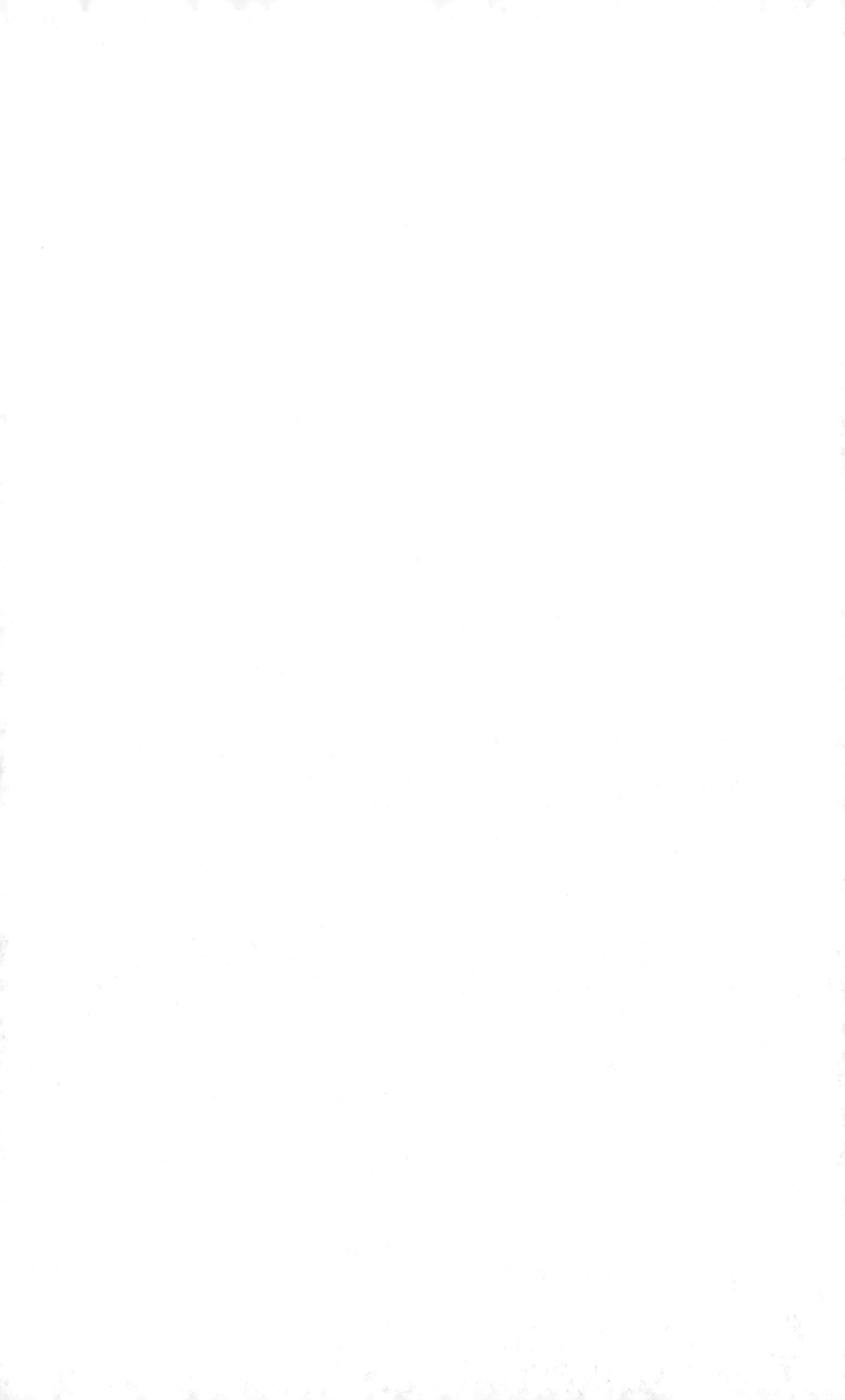

www.ingramcontent.com/pod-product-compliance
Lightning Source LLC
Chambersburg PA
CBHW051555250726
48653CB00004BA/1162